C is for Childhood Cancer

And Other Lessons Cancer Taught Me

Katie Vandrilla

10% of the proceeds of this book will be donated to fight childhood cancer

Dedication

To my family, friends, and teachers—
your support and dedication kept me going when
everything felt uncertain.

To Johnny Depp, whose films continue to give me escape
when I need it most.

And to Lana Parrilla, whose projects help me keep
healing—proof that good can come from broken.

I'm where I am because of you. This is for all of you—
my light in the dark.

Table of Contents

Introduction

I sat in an unyielding chair in the waiting room of my pediatrician's office. A chair that emulated actual plush cushioning but was more plastic meets concrete. My family filled the other three blue and aqua seats adjacent to mine. They surrounded me like a force field, even though they were powerless in protecting me from what we were up against.

The faint but steady aroma of sterile isopropyl alcohol stung my nostrils.

It was the middle of the day on a Wednesday.

My brother was supposed to be at law school.

My dad never missed work and shouldn't have been there.

My mom didn't work on Wednesdays and usually spent the day at home lesson planning for the next day, among other things.

I should have been in school.

We did not belong *there*.

The only other people in the waiting room were babies and toddlers and their parents.

I knew whatever the reason we had to come back, it wasn't good. I mean, how often does a doctor make everyone in a family drop what they're doing in the middle of the week to come *in person* for *good* test results?

Any minute, our lives were about to change.

My palms were sweaty, and my heart was thumping so loudly I could hear it in my ears. With each *thump*, a pulsing throb echoed around my skull.

Eventually, the wooden door which separated the waiting room from the exam rooms opened, and the person who came out read my name off their clipboard.

"Katherine?"

This is it. No going back now.

Together, as a family, we entered the exam room to hear three words no one ever wants to.

"You have cancer."

Those words didn't echo through the room. They didn't need to. They landed like lead—silent, heavy, final.

It's never a good time for cancer to enter your life (and one day, hopefully, there will be a cure).

For me, this came at the start of my junior year of high school when I was sixteen. "*Sweet sixteen*" … when I was diagnosed with leukemia. Just when I should have been figuring out who I was, and what I wanted to do with the rest of my life, I was thrown into a fire I never could have imagined.

While each of my friends was going for their driver's tests, I was going for blood tests.

While they were going on dates, I had dates to keep at the hematology/oncology clinic.

While they were getting their hair done for the next dance, I was getting fitted for my wig.

While they were studying for school, I was studying the potential side effects of my newest medication.

Up to this point, we had lived parallel lives and experiences. Now my life was a tangent, derailing in a different direction.

Each day was a win, as it meant I was still surviving. "Happy Birthday" became a victory song. Each year I got to hear it was another trip around the sun that I knew no one was promised, but I was fortunate enough to get. I *loved* my birthday, and always will because of this. Cancer taught me that getting older is a privilege not afforded to all.

Let me just say here and now, cancer is not something you can out-will. If that were the case, the strongest of the strong would always prevail, and that is unfortunately not so. I have no idea why some survive while others do not. This is something I have questioned time and time again since I was diagnosed, and still don't have an answer to. Particularly each time I lose another friend to the disease. There is absolutely no way that I just "wanted" to survive more than they did, and definitely not even the slimmest chance that I "deserved" to live longer. Survivor's guilt has torn me apart, but I have learned to enjoy each moment I have stolen from fate, and try to make the world a brighter place because I'm here. But let's take a step back.

Before I could get to that kind of reflection, I had to understand what was happening inside me—literally.

It all started with one cell. One cell that decided to change the course of my life. If you didn't know, because you had no good reason to before this point in your life, leukemia begins when the DNA of a developing white blood cell is damaged. Instead of continuing to grow into a functional cell, it begins to multiply uncontrollably, doesn't do what it's supposed to (fight infections), and doesn't die when it's supposed to. Soon, what began as one cell is crowding the bone marrow, which can no longer produce the healthy blood cells it needs to keep the body functioning.

Leukemia is considered a "liquid tumor" because the cells are not a solid mass, but flow freely in the circulatory system. (The free medical knowledge comes as a bonus of going through cancer treatment.)

Everything my life has become, and almost every change it has gone through, can be traced back to that single cell. I spent so much time *resenting* that cell, and my body for not eliminating it. Your body has procedures in place to take care of issues (such as single cells that go astray). Many people have these cells that can flip their lives upside down in the blink of an eye floating around in their bodies. But your body is an incredible machine and takes care of it before you lose the upper hand.

And yet, beyond the biology, there was something far more complicated to untangle: how I felt about all of it. It took me a long time to process and be thankful for that cell and the consequential blessings it has brought to my life.

Yes … you read that correctly.

In my own strange way, I'm thankful for how my life turned out. Cancer included.

At the moment I was diagnosed, it felt like the worst possible thing that could happen to me. Maybe you or someone you love was recently diagnosed with something and feel similarly. That's a perfectly normal response to a life-altering moment. Over time I began to see the bigger picture of my story. I also saw all of the positive aspects of my life which were unforeseen consequences of my diagnosis, such as the lessons the whole experience taught me.

Writing became one of the ways I sorted through it all. I started writing this book for myself. It started as separate essays and was never meant to be read by anyone else (and maybe still won't be … I hope that's not the case … But no matter what, it was worth it). I was trying to process what I had been through since I heard the words "you have cancer." It then got to a point where I thought maybe someone in a similar situation could benefit from reading it. That possibly reading some of my reflections on the lessons I learned could help someone sort through their emotions, recognize something that may be happening in their own journey, or better advocate for themselves. Or maybe cancer has never touched your life, but this book will help you realize some of what I've learned the hard way, such as everyone is fighting their own battle (so be kind to each other).

This memoir is open and honest. If you're reading this, except for the few aspects I ultimately decided to keep private, my life is *literally* an open book (unless you're reading it as an eBook, in which case I don't know if it's technically "open …" My dry sense of humor is my free gift to you).

This book is chaotic at times, because it's about life. *My life*. And no matter how hard you try, you can't make your life seem logical and planned, because that would belong in the fiction section (nothing against fiction; all of my previous written works have been fiction). But this is real … as real as my memory says it is.

It was also a challenge to write because of something many cancer survivors experience: "chemo brain." Do you know how difficult it is to write about moments in your life during which you suffered a form of memory loss? "Chemo brain" (which, ironically, I don't remember if I've explained later …) is a common term to describe any memory or cognitive challenges a cancer patient may experience. This can be short- or long-term and can include symptoms like confusion, memory loss (that was the big one for me), trouble concentrating or paying attention (another one I struggled with), difficulties making decisions, or learning challenges. I have some of these effects lingering to this day, which I have had to learn to live with (not that my family is notorious for having superb memories to start with …).

Reading through drafts of this book, I kept seeing that I wrote the same section or story several times over. I did this because I kept forgetting that I already wrote it. So a good chunk of the time I spent revising this memoir has been going through duplicate stories to see which one was more cohesive or went along with the tone I was aiming for with the overall book. I'm telling you this in case you keep forgetting what you're reading or think something sounds familiar, that's okay! I won't blame you for forgetting something I said or you read (even though everything I have to say is *awesome* …) as long as you don't blame me for repeating myself occasionally.

Some names have been eliminated, but the people who know me I expect to read this book, will know who I'm talking about (*Hi Mom!*).

If you have ever been in my life, at any point, for any length of time, you have affected me. Knowing you has shaped my journey, even if you don't have your own chapter here. If you helped or offered my family assistance when we were in the midst of everything (even if we didn't take you up on it), it meant the world to us. So … Thank you.

I hope you learn something from this book—or at the very least, feel like someone out there gets it. Whatever "it" is for you.

PART ONE

The Beginning:
Diagnosis & Treatment

Chapter 1
Background

Everyone has a story. This is mine.

Before I was diagnosed, I was your perfectly ~~normal~~ … completely ~~average~~ … extremely *weird* teenager. Everyone thinks they're "special," but I have struggled with fitting in my entire life. It always felt as if everyone was better at playing the game of "fitting in" than me.

I was (and anyone who knows me will vouch for me … still *am*) odd. One of my most cherished—and admittedly most unusual—quirks? One of my best friends growing up was (and still is) a toy bunny named Thumper.

Thumper has been with me since my third Easter. When he first came into my life, he had a bit more fluff than he does now. People used to think he was real, and we almost got thrown out of a restaurant once because they thought we'd brought a live rabbit inside.

It took a few years for me to develop the special bond I have with Thumper. But what we formed is nothing short of unique. I never had imaginary friends. I had plush animals who each had their own personalities.

Thumper is one-of-a-kind. My whole family embraced him as a member (and my parents will enthusiastically tell you he's their favorite child). He comes on escapades with us (such as family trips, my bridal shower, my wedding …) and has a children's book series (called *Thumper's Adventures*) based on him.

Thumper makes friends wherever he goes—including people who've met him in person and those who follow his various social media pages from all over the world. It's difficult to explain. You'll just have to meet him one day or check out his Instagram @ThumperExplores.

When I became ill, Thumper was one of my rocks. He was always there and went through everything by my side. I've never felt alone when he's there. Even if some people don't consider him "real," I certainly do. Everyone deserves the kind of comfort having a friend like Thumper provides.

Just like Thumper offered a constant sense of security, so did school—a place where I felt at home, challenged, and inspired. I've always loved school. Since a young age, I planned on becoming a teacher and understood I should get as much out of my education as possible. Probably since my parents sent me to two pre-K programs simultaneously (one I went to "on my own" and the other was taught by my mom). You learn so much in school. Even if you don't remember everything, it opens your mind and your world to new ways of thinking, other experiences, different perspectives from your own, and provides countless opportunities to grow as an individual. I'm lucky I had such a wonderful experience with education and know that not every child is provided with the same opportunities or educators that have a passion for what they do as I did. I just hope that as a teacher myself, I'm doing my part to give future generations an educator who loves their job and subject.

So, yes. I was a teacher's pet. I was one of *those* kids. I *tried* at school … very hard. Nothing I have done in my life has come easy to me. I've had to work my butt off, but I have an intrinsic drive to keep bettering myself and getting the most out of every chance I'm given.

I was also fortunate that my OLDER brother, D.J., was my other best friend growing up. (He was even my man of honor at my wedding.) Many people think I'm older than him, so I wanted to set the record straight. He is OLDER than me. By over five years! Of course we fought. We're siblings. But we have shared countless great times together. I couldn't have asked for a better older brother. D.J. was always there to catch me when I fell … one time literally which saved my life (I keep my Guardian Angel on their toes). He helped shape how I approach relationships—with honesty, loyalty, and a whole lot of humor. And … Did I mention he's older?

As I got into middle school, those values helped me form a friend group that, for the first time, stuck around longer than a school year. Until then, my close friends tended to rotate with my class schedule each year, and we would grow apart the following year when we no longer saw one another daily. But in middle school, I reconnected with someone I had known in pre-K (my "own" class), someone from my girl scout troop, and their other friends. We became close (they were already and welcomed me in), and that bridged the gap into high school when everything became real.

Around that same time, something else "real" happened—at least to me. I discovered one of the truest loves of my life (and my husband knows this): Johnny Depp. That was the year that *Pirates of the Caribbean* came out. My family went to see it in the cinema, and I enjoyed the character of Captain Jack Sparrow. Between the summer when it premiered and December when it came to DVD (Remember those shiny round flat discs?), my family told me Captain Jack Sparrow was the same actor as Edward Scissorhands. *Yeah, right.* One of my weird talents is being good at recognizing actors from one project to another. (Today, I use that gift to try to connect everyone within a few degrees of separation to Johnny ... because ... why not?) My mom then pointed out a normal-looking actor in a film called *Nick of Time* and tried to get me to believe that he, *too*, was Captain Jack Sparrow. And you think *your* parents are crazy ... There was *no way* I could wrap my brain around it. That was *not* the same person. Period. My brother also told me about a fourth film Captain Jack Sparrow "was in." A film I had never watched more than five minutes of because it terrified me after two people were decapitated ... *Sleepy Hollow.* I could not see the connection. I didn't believe it. Clearly my family was insane and lying to me (that was the only logical explanation).

By the time *Pirates of the Caribbean* was getting ready to be released on DVD, I became excited about it and interested in learning more. Like, so interested that I decided to figure out Captain Jack Sparrow's real name and previous work. This was before everyone had the internet at their fingertips … the Stone Age. We were doing a collage of things we liked in English class. I had a catalog with a tiny picture of the DVD cover that I decided to include on my poster. I couldn't even make out the names of the actors in the image (a squint-to-see-how-good-you-can-make-your-eyesight test) and asked my teacher for help. Was his name the one above this face? Something *too small to read* Bloom? Or was it one of the first names?

Something *way too small* Knightley? Or something *are those even letters* Depp? My teacher (aka, 2003's version of Google) eventually helped me figure out his name was Johnny Depp. She asked if I wanted her to blow up his name on the copier to include on my collage. *You can do that? Um, sure.* I liked his character, but now that I knew his name, I thought I liked him more than I realized. Because, that makes sense to a twelve-year-old, right? Little did I know, something was happening inside me. My brother might say that this was the beginning of insanity … I'm not sure I would classify "fangirling" as crazy (as long as you remember that celebrities are real people with rights and lives and deserve privacy … which I totally do).

I went home that night to our family computer, with the hardwired internet (waited several minutes for the earsplitting dial-up as it loaded), and looked up this "Johnny

Depp." *Oh, look at that.* He really *was* Edward Scissorhands. He entirely eluded my uncanny ability to recognize actors across roles—which made him instantly intriguing.

The more I learned, the more fascinated I became. He seemed like such a sweet guy. And not too bad on my preteen hormonal eyes, either. I printed my first pictures of him (again, we didn't have the ability to call images up on our phones whenever we wanted), and the rest is history. I knew this was a love and admiration that was going to last a lifetime. It just felt different than other celebrity "crushes" I'd had. Every day that passed, and the more that I learned about Johnny, the deeper in I was. I'll never forget, about a week or two after my infatuation began, one of my classmates told me to move on; that I would never meet him and probably wouldn't even like him in a few weeks. I have no idea who that kid was, but I've since (over the next 20 plus years) met Johnny twice (and counting) and worked on a book with him. More on Johnny later, but he instantly became a huge part of who I was. Most people who know me can't help but think of me when they see Johnny—which is fine by me. What I didn't realize back then, though, was just how much he'd come to mean in the years ahead.

But life in high school wasn't only about celebrity crushes and awkward growing pains. It was also where I began to explore who I really was—through clubs, classes, and the people who helped shape my future. By high school, I was exceedingly involved in extracurricular activities. If an opportunity presented itself to me, I was going to take it. That same friend from pre-K was in one of those clubs, the robotics team. That was a lot of fun, especially since I have ZERO knowledge of robotics or engineering. But I got to use power tools, which I had always enjoyed, and had many great experiences. Such as traveling to the national competition in Georgia and occasionally getting to drive the robots (well, operating the arm apparatus).

There were a few other clubs I joined—like the school newspaper, Science Club, and Future Teachers—but the one that truly stole my heart (and my time) was the Drama Club. That club had a fall "straight play" (with no music) and would do improv games just about every week after school (and we'd compete once a year against other schools in an improv tournament). In the spring, the music department would run the musical. (I was always in the chorus, as I never exactly learned how to sing.) The Drama Club would also help with the Haunted Mansion nearby in the fall (where we'd get to dress up and scare people). Needless to say, the Drama Club took up much of my free time. And I was very willing to give that time.

But it wasn't just after-school activities that shaped me. One classroom experience, in particular, changed everything about how I saw learning—and myself.

In tenth grade, I took Chemistry. This was a class that my expectations were built up for over the past several years since my brother had taken it. D.J. had an incredible teacher, who my parents had always said would be perfect for me. I'd been rather lucky in terms of science teachers, and it was one of my favorite subjects throughout school. When I received my schedule at the beginning of the year, I skimmed, looking for that name. I would be lying if I said I wasn't initially disappointed that I didn't see my brother's teacher on the list. It was the only name I was checking for, and I didn't even recognize the name that was there. *Oh, well.* This clearly was not going to be what I expected and therefore would have no further purpose to mention ever again. Right? Because when we don't immediately get what we want, it's certainly going to be a horrible experience, because we obviously know what's best for ourselves one hundred percent of the time.

If there was a sarcasm font (Why hasn't someone figured that out yet?), those last few sentences would have used it. Would the teacher I had originally wanted been perfect for me? Probably. I worked with him briefly later down the line, and he is a brilliant and wonderful human I am honored to have had the chance to know. But was the teacher I was assigned better for me? Does that teacher wish he could have swapped me out for any other student so I didn't and don't continue to bother him for however long he lives? Almost definitely.

Chemistry was one of those "life-changing" experiences. It was the first time I really saw the direct payout for my effort and time in studying. Chemistry did not (and still does not) come easily to me. (All … one … of my current students reading this will be confused right now, even though I tell them I struggled.) I had to try very hard to understand the concepts and went for help quite often (which I'm still sorry for how much time all my teachers had to put in to help me master anything, but *hope* it paid off). Then when I would get my grade after an assessment, I actually felt as if I'd accomplished something.

I learned so much in that class. More than just atoms and reactions—it helped me figure out who I wanted to be. One of the biggest things I learned was what I wanted to teach. I had always wanted to become a teacher but couldn't decide what age student or subject was right for me. I also had this idea that teachers of a certain subject knew everything (probably because I have always asked the most specific and random questions about what we were studying, and everyone always seemed to have the answer). My Chemistry teacher explained that teachers don't know everything and are always learning from and along with the students. That is one of those "duh" moments I feel stupid saying I didn't know when I was fifteen. But that helped me realize that I *could* teach whatever I wanted. And Chemistry was going to be that subject. It would be a long road, and I'd have so much to learn, but I was determined. **You can do anything you set your mind to**. For me, succeeding in chemistry was something I had set my mind to.

Everyone deserves a teacher like him at least once throughout their life. I hope I'm half the teacher to my students as he was to me.

His influence didn't stop when the class ended. I really wanted to take AP Chemistry, but my school didn't offer it at the time. At the start of junior year, I went back to visit that teacher. I'd had the revelation that there is no way most teachers can remember all of their students, and it would really stink if someone who had made such a difference in my life forgot about me … so I didn't want to let that happen as long as I was still in the school. He let my friend and me eat lunch in his room. (Just the fact that he gave up his duty-free lunch to spend time with students says a lot.) He told us that AP Chemistry was going to be approved for the following year, and he was going to be teaching it. Of all the AP classes I thought I was going to take at that moment, this was the one I genuinely was excited for.

I was still involved in all my extracurricular activities, and I was, of course, still trying my best in school. I had every intention of following in my brother's footsteps (because everything with us was a competition) and taking all of the Advanced Placement courses I could (essentially like he had done before me). By my junior year, I was in AP Biology and was on track to take Spanish V, Calculus, Physics or the new Chemistry (if it really was going to be offered), and English or U.S. History my senior year—and have a mental breakdown.

In hindsight, that kind of schedule would've been one of the worst decisions I could have made. Mental health wasn't something we talked about much back then, but I now realize that path would've pushed me past my limit. I've since learned to take care of my mental *and* physical health—and that includes knowing when to say no. But to sixteen-year-old "I-know-what's-best" Katie? It sounded like the perfect plan. Start college with a whole semester done? Yes, please.

Or so I thought.

Reality hit quickly. By the end of the first quarter of junior year, I was struggling to keep up with just AP Biology and realizing in Spanish IV that I was nowhere close to approaching fluency. My plans were looking a little shaky, but I would just have to keep pushing. It didn't help that I was starting to become extremely fatigued and losing the drive to do everything. From school work, to staying after for Drama Club, to even eating … (Have I mentioned that I LOVE food? I am one of those "live to eat" people and have trouble relating to the "eat to live" people.) Instead of remaining after school, I was heading home to take naps. Long naps. I hadn't taken those since I was a toddler. I enjoy my sleep but just don't *nap*. After school, I would sit on the couch "just for a minute." My eyes would grow heavy, and before I knew it, I was asleep and losing several hours of consciousness. Then I would sleep the whole night and still be tired in the morning. Something was wrong. And if you ever feel that something is wrong, go get answers. Don't accept "you're fine" if you know deep down you aren't. Trust your gut. I have been blessed with wonderful doctors in my life, but doctors are human. They miss things; they make mistakes. If you think you're sick, get a second opinion when someone tells you you're not.

This was only getting worse, so we knew I should get checked out. My parents must have thought I was depressed or developing an eating disorder. I know we all thought that I could have had mono or the onset of diabetes. We needed answers so I could get better.

My mom drove me in the family van to the pediatrician's office. My physician did a checkup, asked some questions … what doctors do. She had me lie down on the exam table. The sanitary paper crinkled underneath my body. She gently pressed around on my abdomen to feel my internal organs. While her touch should not have been painful, I felt tender. As she moved about and hit my lower left, a shock of discomfort coursed through me, making my face cringe. When she made her way to the right, a similar sensation knocked the wind out of me. She focused on those two areas before having me sit up.

While she didn't say exactly what she was thinking, she didn't like what she felt.

She asked my mom to take me immediately to get bloodwork done. It was almost 5 o'clock, and we said we would go the next day since no place would be open by the time we got there. My doctor wasn't okay with that response. She called the closest blood draw to us, told them we were coming, and requested they wait for us.

We got there right at the time they should have been closing, but the lovely phlebotomists took me in and drew my blood. I remember looking around the office and noticing that there were many indentations in the plush carpet, as if all the furniture had been moved recently. (My favorite show at the time was *Monk*, and that is a detail he would have picked up on if that had been a crime scene … I may watch too much television.)

It was a little difficult to access my veins to collect the blood samples. When the needle pierced my skin, it was as if my vein moved out of the way. Apparently, I have blood vessels as stubborn as I am. The phlebotomist was able to massage my arm and trick the snarky vein into getting pricked. *At least this wasn't a common occurrence I had to endure.* Or so I thought.

Then my mom and I went about the rest of our night as usual. I was uneasy, but still didn't fully grasp that something serious might be happening. The last normal night we ever had. I remember I had a performing arts class at the Bushnell (the performing arts center in Hartford) that evening. I wasn't missing that. My parents had paid for me to take the class, and I knew the value of money and opportunity.

There are moments, or days, in your life where everything changes. Points of no return. You know you can never go back to life before that because everything is about to shift. Details are etched in your memory, more so than usual. We probably have several of these in a lifetime. Good or bad. Shared or individual. This can be on a large or small scale. Like, (especially Americans) do you remember where you were during 9/11 (or maybe you're too young for that and I'm dating myself)? What about what you did leading up to the COVID-19 lockdown (in America, that was March 2020)? My parents remember things such as Martin Luther King Jr.'s "I have a Dream" speech or JFK's assassination. Maybe these references will have to be updated one day. It would be nice if the next large-scale event could be a happy one.

On a smaller scale, I've heard the birth of a child is one that I hope to experience eventually. Your life is now defined, in part, by this moment, as you are a parent. Forever.

For me and my family, one such moment of no return was the 14th of November 2007. It was the morning after my doctor's visit. (My physician had gotten the results the night before, but called my mom in the morning. She wanted to give us one last normal night before our lives changed. I appreciate her decision to wait.) I went to school as I had always done. (I was not one to stay home just because I wasn't feeling 100%.) First period, I had a pre-calculus test. I didn't understand any of the questions. It was as if I had no recollection of ever learning those concepts. Normally, I studied exceptionally hard for assessments and sought out extra help ahead of time if I needed it. I just didn't have the energy that time.

I turned it in mostly blank and left the classroom defeated.

After failing that test … probably the only assessment like that I ever failed, I went to study hall and started to work on my homework. Again, everything I was trying to work on seemed like it was in another language, but I pushed through because that's the only way I knew.

Study halls in my school were paired up with our gym and science classes. It was an odd, but efficient, setup. Science classes had an extra period (or two) a week to build in time for labs, based on the level of the course. Those other "extra" periods you weren't in science, you were in gym some of the year or study hall at other points. I stared out the cafeteria window (which was internal and showed the hallway), and my biology teacher was pointing me out to a secretary. This person had come looking for me and must have checked with my teacher first since this was partially my science period. When someone comes personally looking for you in school, that probably isn't good. I packed up and followed them to the guidance office. That still couldn't be good (not that lovely things don't happen there, but I wasn't even thinking about college yet, which was a big part of what they helped with).

I will never forget walking into my counselor's office. She had been crying. My mom and brother were there. My mom had been crying.

I knew something was wrong.

This definitely wasn't good. It clearly was about what happened at the doctor's, but I was already prepared for either a mono or diabetes diagnosis. These people were overacting … right?

My mom said that my doctor had called, and she wanted to talk about my test results. We had to go to her office immediately, and Dad would meet us there. *Wait … Dad was coming from work (which he never missed)? To talk about mono? Okay …*

Even with everything going on, my brain made a hard turn to something completely unrelated—my part in the school play. I had just recently been promoted to my first decent-sized role. The play was about two weeks away. Silly me, this is what I thought of first. Even dumber than that, I spoke my thoughts (as I often do).

"I don't care if I'm dying, I'm still doing the play."

Oh, boy. I struck a chord with that one, and my guidance counselor's expression is still ingrained in my head to this day. Her face dropped. I thought she was going to burst into tears. I felt horrible and was starting to get nervous.

We left the school and headed to the pediatrician's office. I saw a slip of paper that said "hematology/oncology" and some other letters in the netted basket between the driver's and passenger's seat of the van. Unfortunately … *maybe fortunately* … I had no idea what either word meant at the time. Even though I was in AP Biology, we had been learning about plants, not the medical terms for *blood* and *cancer*.

Before I knew it, we were in the waiting room. Blue is supposedly a calming color. I wondered if they chose blues to decorate the area to comfort the general patient who might feel uneasy about visiting the doctor, or if it was more for moments such as this. When you know your world is about to come crashing down, and perhaps the subtle psychiatry of a soothing color palette was intentional. The calm before the storm.

I was soon in the exam room with my pediatrician and my whole family. She said there was an irregularity in my blood, that there were too many white blood cells. I had leukemia … *cancer*. At that moment, everything stopped. Time froze, and I wished so hard that I had either misheard, or this was a dream, or there was a mistake. Then time resumed.

So that is why everyone had been crying. And now, I was crying, too, and I didn't care to hide it. Hot tears were streaming down my face.

My doctor asked me what questions she could answer for me. The main ones I remember were if I would lose my hair and if I would die. She assured me that the survival rate was decent for that type of cancer, and I'd get the best treatment available, but I would lose my hair. I would be going to the children's hospital in Hartford (thankfully not very far away) and meeting with the doctor who would take over my care to try to cure the leukemia.

What happened next was a blur. She said we had to pack, as I could be in the hospital for up to a month for the first stay. I had never been overnight in the hospital and felt okay (not month-long-stay ill). The idea of being there a month sounded horrible and didn't make sense. I think I went home and packed (which my family helped me with), and we went up to Connecticut Children's Medical Center (CCMC) together. Two "items" that became staples in my hospital stays: my toy bunny Thumper and my purple fuzzy slippers (which my brother called "Muppet feet").

Our destination was a clinic called "2J." We waited in *that* waiting room (I guess that's why it's called that) until it was our turn. My parents were given a stack of forms to complete. Based on the amount of paper, they were either filling out our entire family's medical history, or being asked to read the receptionist's screenplay.

That room had the same isopropyl alcohol aroma as my pediatrician's office. As if the room and all of its contents had been sanitized to the point you could safely lick the floor without getting sick … any sicker than you already were. I could tell that this was a scent that was going to follow me.

There were different families that came and left, and various doctors and nurses that came through while we waited. I sat on my navy-blue chair, hoping there was some mistake. Certainly, I didn't have *cancer*. The people who took my blood samples must have put the wrong label on it because it was closing time and they were tired, or someone must have read my results incorrectly.

Something … Anything.

There was an honest mistake made and any moment someone would figure it out, call us, and tell my family we could go home. Back to our regular lives.

This is what you call the denial phase. I'm no expert in the phases of grief/trauma, but I understand that one.

This isn't happening.

Maybe it's all a dream and I'll wake up in the comfort of my bed any second.

I took another look at the other families and kids in the waiting room. Much more of a variety than at the pediatrician's. It was still the middle of the day. We all belonged elsewhere. Those other kids should be in school. This was not where they should be if they were having a normal, healthy childhood. Did they even understand what was going on and that they were having their childhood interrupted? This wasn't fair to them or their family.

As I was looking around, I saw a sign about Alex's Lemonade Stand. I knew that charity raised money for childhood cancer research, so this was the perfect spot. After reading the sign, I learned who Alex was. She was an incredibly strong, kind, and optimistic young girl who wanted to help other kids with cancer. (She tragically had cancer most of her life and passed away from it when she was only eight.) Alex was treated at CCMC and started her lemonade stand to raise money so the doctors could help other kids with cancer.

I was crying again.

Here I was, selfishly grieving for myself, while a child half my age had literally made lemonade out of the lemons she was handed, just to help others. However long it took, I had to see the world more like this inspiration and make something positive out of this situation.

Still, my mind kept wandering. That's when I saw a doctor come through a side door and enter the locked doors of the clinic with his badge. *Wait ... You couldn't get into the doors ... Was this a prison?* I had this feeling that he was going to be my doctor. No reason other than instinct. He didn't look at us, speak, or do anything differently than everyone else that was moving about.

When it was finally our turn, they called my name and brought us to the locked doors. The nurse tapped her ID badge on a reader with a steady red light on it. There was a singular *beep* as the light changed to green, followed by a strong *click* resonating from the doors themselves. In a swift motion, the nurse opened the doors and escorted us inside the clinic.

They took my vitals, for the first of a million times. This included your typical height and weight, blood pressure, oxygen reading, and temperature. We fumbled through this, as I was not quite sure what body part to offer for which device they were sticking on me. Eventually, this would be more of a dance: my shoes would be off by the time I got to the scale, and my arm and opposite index finger would be extended for the O_2 sensor and blood pressure sleeve by the time I was seated in the chair. It's incredible what can become routine when you had never even known the process existed before a certain moment in time.

I struggled to get my shoes back on (in time I would just carry these with me from the vitals chair to my room), and we were led to our own private exam room. Now I understood why we had waited so long. There were only a few exam rooms in this clinic; they clearly had to expand for the number of patients they were seeing each day (which they did over the next few years as they moved upstairs to "5A"), and they were setting us up for what felt like was going to be a while. They showed us how to work the TV and tried to make us as comfortable as possible. Because I was *totally* in the mood to get comfortable at that moment. I was staring at the door, waiting for someone to come in and let us know about the big mix-up.

The room felt small and a little too quiet after the hustle of the waiting area. But inside, I soon realized it wasn't just the room that was cramped—my mind was, too. One after another, people came in and out, filling the space with names, faces, and information I could barely keep up with.

Each of them had a lot to say. Not one of them mentioned the mistake I was anticipating nor sent us home. I don't remember most of what happened over this period of time. I was overwhelmed by all of the new information they were giving us. They were talking about what to expect during treatment, and how things could go depending on the type of leukemia I had. *Wait, there's more than one type of leukemia? That's a shame for people who actually have it. Can I leave now?*

I do remember the doctor I had seen earlier coming in and introducing himself as my oncologist (I had learned by this point that was someone who treats cancer). Let's call him Doctor P. He went through the procedure I would have the following day. I'm not even going to pretend I understood what he was saying. Let's blame the denial, and that this really didn't matter to me. I did catch that something they would do the following morning would not only tell them what type of leukemia I had, it would set me on a treatment plan. He explained the different treatment schedules, but they all averaged around two and a half years. *Wow. So glad I won't have to do that!* That's a long time for anyone, let alone a sixteen-year-old. He said they would put something under my skin to make accessing my veins easier. I certainly misunderstood this part. I was thinking they would slide a needle under my skin and keep it there during whatever treatments they thought they were going to have to give me. My mom had talked about something along those lines before for a blood test she had done. I had almost no experience with blood being drawn or needles. Basically, just what they did the previous day to get the sample to set this whole misunderstanding in motion and the occasional prick/shot at the pediatrician's office. *Cool. Good talk. Sorry I'll never see you again, as you seem like a nice person, Doctor P.*

After Doctor P finished explaining the upcoming procedure—or at least trying to—the door opened again. This time, Christine, a Child Life Specialist, came in to help me understand what was ahead in a very different way. I feel very bad for my reaction to her and what I called her for the next few months as I was learning her name. (Names are difficult for me without being pumped full of chemicals that affect your memory.) She came in with a doll named Lily to "explain" the procedure I would have the next morning. (I later learned that the doll's gender could be changed so any child would be able to relate to it.)

It started quite normally. She showed me two variations of what might stick out of my skin: A Hickman or a Port-o-catheter ("port"). The only odd part was it was sticking out of the doll's chest instead of its arm like I had expected. Okay. Then Christine pulled the front of the doll's chest off to show me what under the skin looked like. That is when I almost passed out, and my brother and dad freaked out a little. In the doll's chest was a tube connecting to its heart. Christine explained how the device worked. It led directly into the arteries at the heart so medicines got around the body quickly, and blood could be drawn efficiently without compromising small veins. I was completely caught off guard. I hadn't realized that this "procedure" was actually surgery—and the doll's chest being opened up made it terrifyingly real. Suddenly, what had seemed like a simple needle under my skin felt like something much, much worse. Now I had questions. Apparently, my mom did comprehend that this was going to be a surgery, but none of the rest of us had.

Now that I was on the same page as everyone with what the true goal of this "procedure" was, I needed it explained from the top. I had never had a surgery before and wasn't ready to be cut open like a frog or worm in science class. The surgery sounded simpler than the doll made it appear, but I'd be lying if I didn't tell you that I was traumatized by the toy and the "Scary Doll Lady" (sorry, Christine) for some time. I understand that the doll is educational and a great tool, but it was one of those moments in my life that scared the crap out of me. Christine is a lovely person, and I got to know her in a much less terrifying environment later, known as "teen group." More on that later.

Needing a distraction, I turned to Harry Potter 2 on the PlayStation—anything to keep my mind off what was coming. But soon enough, it was time to stop pretending this was just another day. I was admitted to the hospital for what would be my first of many stays at CCMC and moved up to my private room. I'm grateful that they had the facilities to give each patient in that ward ("MS8") their own room and also allow an adult family member to stay overnight. That made so many nights easier: being in my own space and almost always with someone from my family. I never even went to sleep-away camp, so being on my own for the first time in a hospital would have been difficult.

Up on MS8, we met more people, but I don't remember much from that part of the day … It had been a lot to take in. I did remember my first nurse's name. We became close, but I didn't have her for long. I also met a doctor who had leukemia as a child. She was really nice and gave me hope I'd make it to the other side.

Once I was settled in my room, I found myself reaching for the phone. I needed to hear a familiar voice—someone who might understand what I was going through. I picked up the plastic receiver with its curly-Q cord that tethered it to the wall, and I called one of my best friends. We used to talk for hours on the phone. Remember when people actually used to call people on the phone? We would time our conversations and see how long we could go. We easily hit over two hours. He had a procedure done a few years before, and I thought he would be the best to talk to about all of the thoughts going on in my head. I had been there for him at that time in his life, and he was there for me during mine. I'm very appreciative that my friends at that point in my life were what I needed and were there. Growing up and growing apart is inevitable for most high school friends, but I will never take for granted how they supported me through the hardest parts of treatment.

When I called him, I didn't quite know what to say. I think I asked him if he had been given a port when he had his surgery. (I still didn't quite understand this was because I was going to need it over a long period of time and not just for a short hospital stay.) He had no idea what that was, and I explained it. (I'm sure I was *100% accurate* with *that* description …) *How do you tell someone you have a critical illness that could potentially end your life?*

He was rightly confused, and eventually I ended up blurting out that I had cancer and was in the hospital. The silence of his response was deafening. And so began my life of making people feel uncomfortable when I unloaded my struggles on them. He rushed up to the hospital to visit that night with his mom. Everyone deserves a friend like he was at least one time in their life.

His mom was an incredible warrior for me during treatment. It would take ages for the hospital pharmacy to get the medicines the doctors ordered, but when you're dealing with the pain and side effects of something like cancer, time is of the essence. I'll never forget one time, when I was waiting for a "miracle mouthwash" because my mouth was full of mouth sores and even water felt like razor blades in my mouth. (The mouthwash would provide a temporary numbing, so you would be able to eat something without the excruciating pain.) My friends had come up for dinner, and I couldn't bear eating anything. She got me the miracle mouthwash within a few minutes. Everyone should have someone like her fighting in their corner for them. Don't get me wrong. My parents and brother were always there fighting for me and helping me get what I needed. This woman was just a tad feistier that particular day.

As I settled into hospital life, one of the first things I got used to was my IV pole—my newest, and very clingy, companion. My friend and I walked around the locked hospital wing (where you could only enter if someone let you in) with my IV pole in tow. I named him Dexter. You have to be familiar enough with a device that is connected to you 24/7 for possibly the next month to be on a first name basis with them. He was "Dexter" because the saline drip he was giving to keep me hydrated had dextrose in it. I knew that was a sugar and thought that was odd. Science has always fascinated me, and I wanted to know more about what was being administered to me. So began my journey of learning as much as I could about the medicines and treatments ahead.

If there's one thing I learned early on: be an active part of your medical treatment. Ask questions. Know what's going into your body so you can take part in the decisions.

On that walk with my friend (not Dexter), we had a heavy—and probably awkward—conversation, punctuated by long stretches of deafening silence. He asked if I wanted him to tell our other friends. I said yes. That made it much easier on me; I didn't have to see their reactions. Not many sixteen-year-olds have faced their own mortality, and not everyone has come to terms with the fact that someone their own age can die. Everyone reacts differently to that. Even adults don't always take that news well. Over the next few years, I encountered all sorts of responses when people saw me. Some thought my cancer was contagious. Others thought I was going to die in front of them. Some didn't want to touch me. Others didn't want to see me, because they couldn't face looking at me sick. If I could avoid some of those moments, it made things a tad smoother for me. I didn't have the energy to comfort others struggling with my illness. I had to focus on coping with my own mortality first.

Thankfully, my friend took on the job of telling everyone at school for me—including our Chemistry teacher from the previous year. Well, that was probably the moment I could have stopped worrying about that teacher ever forgetting me. I know as a teacher, whenever a student (that you know of) has a critical illness, those tend to be students you can't forget.

Over that first week, the Drama Club called me from their classroom, all excited on the phone. *Seriously* … talking on the phone (without seeing faces) was still a thing! It felt so good to hear their voices.

But I also had to deliver the hardest news: I had to tell the director that I couldn't be in the production opening in two weeks. I really didn't want to say it—or to drop out. I'd never backed out of a play commitment before, or since. Hence why right before I learned I was sick, I said "even if I'm dying, I'm doing the play." And even after initially learning about my diagnosis, I was under the delusion I was still going to be in the show. Deciding I had to drop out of the performance felt like I was being defeated. My mind was not going to win over matter this time.

Soon, everyone knew me as "the kid with cancer." Even people and teachers I'd never met before. It was … spooky. I felt like an undeserved celebrity—I hadn't done anything special. They called me "inspiring," and while I get it, my low self-esteem (Don't we all have this as teenagers?) made me question it. How was I inspiring? Just for living? Isn't that what we're all trying to do? I didn't ask to get cancer, and was dealing with it the only way I knew how. In fact, I was a little disappointed in myself for not being more positive the whole time. Between the chemically imbalanced emotions, and just having a difficult time staying optimistic, I felt more like a Debby Downer than an Inspiring Ina. (Okay, I may have just made that name up.)

The morning after my diagnosis, I wasn't allowed to eat or drink anything. Normally, that would have been a huge deal—I LOVE food—but I'd barely had an appetite for over a month anyway. Trying to process everything from the day before didn't help.

They want your stomach empty when you're being sedated ("put to sleep"), because your body's reflexes do not work the same way when you're under. If you have any food (or even liquids) in your stomach, there's a risk you may throw up, bringing them back into your throat. If that happens, it could get into your lungs and not only make it difficult to breathe, but can permanently damage your lungs … *What a pleasant thought.*

For reasons unknown, my surgery kept getting pushed back. That happens. There were probably more important or emergency situations that needed the operating room before me. That was fine by me. *Still a slight chance someone might call this all off anyway, right?*

Eventually, it was my turn.

My memories of the next part are quite limited. They explained everything before the procedure to make sure we had no questions. (That was something everyone at the hospital was great about: educating you and giving you a chance to ask questions.) I know my mom went with me into the operating room, to stay until I was out, and the doctors had me count backward from one hundred as they put a mask on me to start the anesthesia process. It was very bright in the OR.

One hundred … I inhaled deeply, knowing that these were the last real moments of life as I knew it. There was no going back. I would wake up (God willing) with an official diagnosis of which leukemia I really did have. No more hope of a mistake … Unless someone bursts in RIGHT NOW TO STOP THIS!

Ninety-nine … I hoped I'd survive this. Surgery, and cancer. I didn't even want to think about what would happen to my parents and D.J. if I didn't.

Ninety-eight …

The next thing I remember was waking up in the recovery room. Sore. But alive. On the right side of my chest, was a bandage covering the incision and a 1.5-inch needle that was stuck deep within the port like a pin cushion. I had a brand new (because *used* would be gross) port-a-catheter (or "portacath," or "port," also known as a "central line" … you get the idea … there's numerous names for it). I'm actually amazed I didn't personally name mine, as I tended to name lots of inanimate objects, especially ones that would be a part of me for a few years. Wow … how dare I be so inconsiderate to not even name it …

My port placement went well. I also had had a bone marrow aspiration (that is where your hip bone is drilled for bone marrow like it's an oil rig) and a spinal tap, aka "lumbar puncture" or "LP" (which is where a needle is inserted in between your lower vertebrae to get a sample of your spinal fluid … more of my trauma and healing surrounding those later). During the lumbar puncture, my first dose of chemotherapy was administered. "Intrathecal" (given into the spinal column) methotrexate. The purpose of this was to prevent any leukemia cells from crossing the blood-brain barrier (a difficult barrier to cross, but dangerous once it has been breached).

Both fluids (I honestly had never thought much about their existence, let alone imagined they would be taken from my body) were tested for leukemia cells (and what type of cells were present). The results of those labs would send me down the rest of my treatment plan (which would eventually be kept in a giant green binder, complete with all other tests, records, and notes).

I was soon wheeled in my bed through double doors that led to special elevators and taken back up to my own hospital room. Later, we heard the results of the tests.

I did have leukemia. That was not a shock at this point.

Specifically, I had Acute Lymphoblastic Leukemia, also known as ALL. In my bone marrow, there were about 93% blasts. Blasts are white blood cells that are dysfunctional and underdeveloped. Instead of doing their designated job, they multiply uncontrollably, which crowds the bone marrow. This prevents the production of healthy cells important for survival (such as red blood cells, platelets, and normal white blood cells). The buildup of blasts in the bone marrow leads to infections, anemia and bleeding (and if left untreated … death). Most leukemia patients start with between 90 and 95% blasts in the marrow. The goal is to have it down to less than 0.1% by the end of four weeks. (Which is technically considered remission. However, as it's not detectable under that amount, and since even one cancer cell can keep multiplying out of control, treatment continues.) I was at that goal in about two weeks, but not without my share of side effects. (We discovered almost two years later that I was essentially being overdosed by several of the chemotherapies because of an enzyme I lacked that should have helped metabolize the medicines quicker.) But … I'm ahead of myself.

The first hospital stay should have been about a week. I was there for six days. I made up the extra hospital time later.

I was home for Thanksgiving. That must have made it nicer for my family because we had lost my grandfather Halloween the previous year. If I had been in the hospital, it would have been like losing a family member two consecutive Thanksgivings. It made the dinner easier to be thankful for, although just being alive to eat it was enough.

I was back in the hospital the following week. In fact, that became a regular routine of mine. I would be out one week, back in the next. It did not even have to be for something serious. If I went in for my weekly appointment with a fever, I had to stay. Any temperature of 100.5 Fahrenheit twice in a half hour, or 101 at all, won me a one-way ticket onto CCMC MS8 (eighth floor).

There were no cancer cells found in my spinal fluid. All in all, that was a decent place to be with a leukemia diagnosis. The survival rate at the time was estimated to be about 90%. That's still 1 of 10 kids not surviving, but relatively, that was a high survival rate compared to other childhood cancers. Because of my gender, age, and type of leukemia, I was locked in for two and a half years of treatment. If I had been born male, I would have had three and a half years. I had to start looking at every win that I could find, and those results had a lot going in my favor. Did that mean it was smooth sailing from that point? Ha! No. Did it mean that I didn't come at all close to being that 1 of 10 who didn't make it? Absolutely not. But I had to hold on to how fortunate I was.

I chose to participate in a clinical study—hoping that my experience could help improve treatments for others. Though I faced many side effects and don't recall if I stayed in the study until the end, I hold on to the hope that something valuable was learned from my journey, even if it's through the pages of this book. Because no survival rate, no matter how high, feels good enough when a child still loses their battle with cancer. And surviving cancer is never truly the end. The treatments that save lives can leave scars—sometimes invisible, sometimes lifelong. That's why we must keep pushing forward, improving every aspect of cancer care, especially for kids.

Chapter 2
Treatment

Disclaimer: My journey started a long time ago. I'm hopeful a lot of progress has been made since, but know we have a ways to go.

In life, you do what you have to do. And when you're thrown a curveball such as a life-altering diagnosis, you can easily fall into a "new normal," complete with routines you never imagined, if that's what it takes to survive.

The hospital I was treated at (CCMC) was designed with kids in mind—bright colors, friendly animal themes, and rounded corners to avoid anything scary. If I hadn't been sick, I might have found it a comforting place. But unfortunately, the feelings I had while there—pain, fear, exhaustion—became inseparable from the hospital itself. Being there meant feeling awful, and I wanted out, always. I correlated feeling the worst with being in the hospital and wanted to do anything to get out whenever I was there.

My family was amazing, ensuring I spent as few evenings alone as possible. (I could probably count on one hand the number of nights I spent alone.) But since, while you're there, you are already feeling awful, all you want to do is go home. The smells, machines, bright lights, and constant vitals being taken remind you that you are not well … As if you needed any reminders.

At the hospital, there was the security of knowing there were professionals right there who could answer our questions. I would keep a journal with me, to write down any question or note I wanted to discuss with the next doctor or nurse who came by (so I wouldn't forget, especially since I was suffering from "chemo brain"). When I was home, a cloud of uncertainty followed me everywhere. All aches, each bloody nose (which I had NEVER experienced before), every bruise, anything that had never happened before, tossed up red flags that terrified me to death. *What if this was a sign of something huge? What if this was the start of the end?* I, and my family, needed to be told that something was normal, or at least a known side effect.

I had an incredible talent of getting almost every possible side effect of my medications, and not only the common ones. For a cancer with a high survival rate, I kept everyone on their toes. I will never forget at the end of treatment, a few people in my inner circle at the hospital mentioned how they were relieved that I made it through. I was certain they said that to all of their patients, but it really stuck with me. I had a few close calls. No one wants to see anyone die of cancer. And no one should ever have to lose to cancer. Everyone who works with cancer patients is a hero. I couldn't get close to so many people who won't make it to the other end.

My port made IV access or blood draws much easier … once I knew what to expect. The first time I went to the clinic, after my initial hospital stay when the port was placed, I had a bit of a panic attack when the nurse went to access it. The port already had a needle in it when I had woken from the surgery, and I didn't think much … or anything … of it. I didn't reason that they would have to access it once they had removed the original needle (which is its own interesting sensation—the pulling of the needle out of the port like a cork out of a bottle … a bottle that's buried in and a part of your chest wall). So the nurse took a giant needle (okay, it was only between 1.5 and 2 inches long … but that's much longer than you think when they are going to shove it into your chest) and came awfully close to my face with it. My vision filled with sparkly yellow stars, and I almost passed out.

I'm not proud of that reaction. There were small children having their port accessed with no issue, and I was a teenager having a fit. The nurse was incredible, talked me down and explained it to me (and that there was *no* other option, no matter how much I begged), and allowed me to compose myself. When they tried again, it went better. The actual inserting of the needle was not that bad. It was a bit of a prick (a bit more sensitive if your body is still healing from the placement procedure). You then feel the needle disappear into the cushion of the port but can tell it's still inside of you. Once the needle is set, it's fine. You could even use a numbing cream on the area ahead of time. I didn't use that more than once or twice, because it didn't make too much of a difference. The cream was messy, had to go on your skin long before being accessed to take effect, and the needle still had to go into you. For me, it wasn't so much the prick of the needle as it was the sight of it coming toward my face and chest. And closing my eyes didn't help, because I *needed* to watch.

If the needle was going to stay in, they'd dress it with bandages to protect it from popping out and keep the opening in your flesh clean and covered. The nurse then had to do a saline flush of the port to get the line ready to use. This is a clear solution (basically salt water), and I would immediately smell salt in my nose and taste it. It was such an odd experience. Some nurses would validate, and others would try to tell me I wasn't actually having the sensation … I was. From there, blood could be drawn back for testing. (The first bit would always be "thrown out" since there was saline mixed with it.) Medicines like chemotherapies could also be injected from syringes. I remember a bright red one that would be administered this way: doxorubicin. Or a hydration IV could be hooked up. Often, it was a combination of all of these. Whenever the port was no longer going to be used for the time being, it was flushed again with saline, then given a heparin lock. The heparin was a yellow liquid which would keep the line from clotting inside, so it was ready to use the next time. (After this step was when the needle could be removed.)

The port was essentially a pin cushion, with tubing that ran directly into my heart. As I mentioned, the cushion area made being accessed super easy … to nurses who knew how to use one. When we were able to use the port, it meant it would be smooth sailing. Unless I had to take a trip to the emergency room, in which case there was rarely a nurse who had ever seen a port before. (That's not their fault, as ports are not super common.) I sometimes miss it now that it's no longer a part of me. I have tiny, stubborn veins (like the rest of me), so any blood test is a challenge for the phlebotomist. I'm also a little bummed they wouldn't let me keep my port when it was removed. It was a biohazard or *whatever*. It was a part of me for almost three years. We went through so much together. (Technically so much went *through* the port.) But I will always have the scar from where they opened me up to insert, and then remove, it. At first, I was ashamed of the scar. Now, I wear it with pride. It's a badge of honor that says, "Hey world, look what I've survived!"

If you've ever had an IV line connected to you, it eventually feels like a part of you—an extension of your circulatory system. Fluids travel through the line just as they do through your veins, until the two feel indistinguishable. Your body can also easily be tricked into giving fluids up through this same route, as blood is often drawn from the line when you are in the hospital.

Spending so much time with an IV pole, you learn its quirks—how far the cord reaches before needing to be unplugged, how it moves as you walk, and which wheels stick or roll smoothly. It's like driving a shopping cart with a mind of its own. Some move smooth as butter. Some pull to one side as you roll them. Others have a wheel that won't touch the ground, or a sticky wheel and won't make turns. You learn how to drive it. It's an extension of your arm, and you don't go anywhere in the hospital without it. If you forget or try, you feel the tug on the needle when the line gets stretched to its limit, and you're reminded with the pinch that you're tethered to a pole.

Just as the IV line becomes an extension of you, you also learn to tune out the regular interruptions of having your vitals taken—blood pressure, temperature, oxygen levels, and more. While I was in the hospital, vitals would happen every four hours. Overnight, they would sometimes … maybe all the time … leave the blood pressure cuff on so all they had to do was connect it to the machine and take the reading (instead of moving your arm to position it correctly to get the band around it). I got used to sleeping through the vitals checks—usually. But one night, after being woken up twice for blood pressure readings, I finally asked why they needed to check so many times in a row. It was one of those seemingly random times that my levels were inexplicably horrible, and they were trying to get another reading until it was better. I don't know if you've ever had your blood pressure taken, but the cuff squeezing your arm like a clingy toddler holding on to their parent for dear life doesn't exactly calm me (or my blood pressure). So that, on top of being woken from my slumber, wasn't going to help my high levels. I can't quite blame them, though. Whenever they would take my temperature and it was over the threshold that was acceptable (100.5 °F), I would want them to try again as I willed my body into cooling off. That never worked, but I still attempted it.

During one hospital stay, I was on a heart monitor when I started feeling stressed. I asked the person I was talking to to stop aggravating me, but they didn't. Soon, the alarms went off, and staff rushed in to check on me. I was fine once I calmed down.

At the end of treatment, before my port removal surgery, I was asked to sign a living will. I don't recall signing one before, since I was a minor and my parents handled those decisions. Even though the removal of a central line is considered a minor procedure, the gravity of doing my first living will hit home. At any point, things could have ended vastly different.

Did I want to be resuscitated? Did I want to be put on artificial life support?

This was in case anything went wrong, of course. But these were conceivable outcomes, or else they wouldn't have been asked.

I went into the operating room in astoundingly different condition than I had two and a half years beforehand. This time, my hair was growing back (instead of about to fall out), and my outlook on life was night and day compared to what it had been in November of 2007. I had been through hell, but this was the last major part of it. Afterwards (hopefully), I would only have follow-up care. That final procedure was the result of years of treatment working exactly as it was meant to. But reaching that point meant enduring what chemotherapy does best—breaking your body down in order to build it back up.

Chemotherapy attacks all fast-growing cells—including healthy ones like hair follicles and blood cells. As I've mentioned, in leukemia, immature white blood cells flood the bloodstream, crowding out healthy cells. Chemo works to reduce these cancerous cells but also lowers healthy white blood cells, platelets, and red blood cells. This means frequent blood transfusions are necessary when "counts" get too low, in order to keep the body functioning. (Because the body needs to be functioning in order to fight for its life.) During my first year, I had around 40 transfusions. Low hemoglobin meant red blood cell transfusions; low platelets meant platelet transfusions to keep my body working. If you have other forms of cancer, there are medicines that can be given to boost your white blood cell counts to help your bone marrow produce more, which keeps you more able to fight off infections. With leukemia, you shouldn't get those treatments because it would encourage the cancer cells to multiply. It was the first time I realized blood could be separated into components and transfused individually, rather than always as "whole blood." (That may be a naive and obvious misconception I had, but one I had never really had to think about until I needed transfusions to keep my body alive.)

I did fine with the red blood cell units, but they took a long time to infuse (about 4 hours per bag, and sometimes I needed more than one back-to-back). If I was lucky and well enough to leave after the infusion, this was able to be done as an outpatient visit. Otherwise, it was done while I was inpatient or could be part of the reason for being admitted. Some of the times I was healthy enough (other than having dangerously low hemoglobin), I went from what would have been short clinic visits, to several hours to accommodate the transfusion. I will always remember going in on New Year's Eve for an appointment, and my levels were so low that I needed two units of blood. That is eight hours, if started immediately. But you had to wait for your counts to come back from the lab to realize you needed the transfusion, then had to wait for the blood to be ordered and arrive before it could be started. Because of this, I ended up ringing in the new year overnight at the hospital. (I was checked in so I would have a room and was able to leave in the morning.) That was an interesting experience. My aunt came up to visit. Visiting hours ended at 8 pm, and we tried breaking the rules that night because it was New Year's Eve. I think she was able to make it until about 10 pm before we got caught and she had to leave. I felt bad (a small part for breaking the rules, but mostly that she didn't get to stay and "celebrate" with us). It was cool to see the fireworks over the city of Hartford at midnight, though. Because we were on the eighth floor, we had a great view of the city from the windows. That is a year I will never forget. I also didn't know how many more New Year's Eves I would see, so I held on to that one as tightly as I could. My resolution was to do whatever I could to make it through the year.

Red cells weren't the only thing I needed help with. Platelets were another story entirely. Whenever I needed platelets (which looked like a bag of freshly pressed apple juice and fortunately only took about 20 or 30 minutes to infuse), I had an allergic reaction. At least it was an uneventful one where I just developed hives everywhere. It was also an easy fix: I just had to take Benadryl before a platelet transfusion from that point on. *Ah ... the powers of modern medicine.*

Benadryl didn't just come in handy for transfusions. It would later play a critical role in one of the scariest reactions I had during treatment—something we never saw coming. I had a liquid medication that I was to take at the onset of my migraines. We somehow missed the instruction that it should be taken with Benadryl. To be fair, treating migraines wasn't as life or death important as getting every step of the chemotherapies correct. And everyone in my household was under the impression that taking Benadryl was *optional.* After a dose or two of the medicine without the Benadryl ... we learned it was quite necessary each time.

I don't remember the time frame between taking the medicine and what happened next. The migraine must have been mostly better by that time, because I don't recall the throbbing of my head on top of what happened to the rest of my body (but, honestly, I could have blocked it out to prioritize what I needed to focus on because I was in panic mode). I was lying on the couch, and my joints (particularly my fingers, neck, and jaw) decided to go slowly, but forcefully, in directions they were not designed to. At first, when the movements were new and mild, it was slightly interesting (in the notion that I had zero control over them, but it wasn't immediately a huge concern …).

I told my mom about it and showed her what was happening. At that point, the movements were still slight, and I could have been moving my body that way on my own (if I was faking … but why would I want to take an extra trip to the hospital, especially when I had only recently gotten home?). My mom immediately knew something wasn't right. The joint contortions kept getting worse and more pronounced (a step down from what Vecna did to his victims in *Stranger Things*), so we called the doctor and ended up in the hospital shortly afterward.

By the time we got to the hospital, any amusement I originally found in the situation had long disappeared. By this point, I was terrified, and sore. I was worried that my joints would go too far and that something was going to break. That was the surface level, immediate concern. As it was, the bones in my fingers were trying to bend from the top joint and spread far apart from one another. My jaw was moving so far horizontally, it felt like any farther and it would snap off (likely dislocate first, but breaking was a definite possibility). I was trying to combat the wrong directional movements by doing everything in my power to force the joints in the opposite direction they were moving. I tried to keep them as in line as possible. This was tiring and made them ache even more than being slammed in the odd positions already had (but again, I was trying to protect my joints by not allowing them to keep moving beyond the planes they were attempting to).

The deeper level concern was *what was causing this? Was I going to be okay?*

Thinking maybe it was a stroke, the doctors did an MRI. Telling someone who has zero control over their joints to "lie still" … yeah right. Of course I kept moving (without being able to tell my joints what to do), but they got enough of what they needed.

After an MRI and an anxious wait, the results came back.

I was fine. *What?!*

Don't get me wrong. I was absolutely relieved that they didn't find something horrendous on the MRI. I was half expecting it to reveal my worst nightmare. But if I was fine, why was my body trying to rip itself apart?

Through a bit of detective work, the doctors and nurses realized the root cause was the interaction of the medication. They asked me if I had taken Benadryl. (At this point, I don't remember that having been instructed at all … let's blame chemo brain on it.) They went over that the medicine could cause the reaction I experienced if I took it without the Benadryl. *Um … okay. I personally would have led with that in the first place when it was prescribed, but I am not a pharmacist.*

I only ever took the medicine with Benadryl from that point … which wasn't long. I quickly asked for an alternative to be found, because knowing what could happen without the Benadryl was unnerving. What else was it capable of doing, even *with* the Benadryl?

As if the medications and their risks weren't enough to worry about, we were also given clear warnings about other things to avoid. We were told that I should stay away from what most parents worry their teenage child will get into: recreational drugs, alcohol, and sex. Now, I was basically your poster child for boring, follow-the-rules kid anyway. But now you tell me that the *extra* (because I was already on a whole lot of what was considered "recreational," but I needed them for medicinal purposes) drugs or alcohol could damage my organs beyond repair and compromise my survival? Or that if I contracted *anything* during intercourse, it could kill me? Yeah … at sixteen, I already wasn't into those things, but that put the kibosh on even the smallest idea of rebelling in that way … Not that I had the energy to or would even find someone interested in touching a cancer patient the way I looked, anyway. (I was *so* fun at parties, even going into college. But, I have no regrets. I probably would have stayed that course anyway. I was safe, I was happy with my choices, and my parents were also happy. There is more than one way to have fun. And no one should force you into doing something you're not comfortable with.)

As we learned more about how chemo affected the body, we also realized that *any kind* of bleeding could be dangerous—especially in my case. Like a large portion of the population, I had a monthly period. Even a normal cycle became a threat when my platelet counts were low—

sometimes so low I would bleed *as if* I had my period, even when I wasn't menstruating. To manage this risk, they essentially induced a temporary menopause that lasted two and a half years. I got a monthly birth control shot known as Depo (easy to remember, because I called it "Depp-o"), which looked and felt like milk being injected into my arm. But it worked—my period stopped almost immediately and didn't return for nearly three years.

Of course, medically pausing your body's natural cycle doesn't come without side effects. I'm not sure how much you know about the menstrual cycle, but it's supposed to happen until you come across that point in your life when you go through natural menopause (or are pregnant). That was how the body was designed. Even naturally hitting menopause creates changes to the body and hormones and fun stuff like that. I had the pleasure of experiencing (what I assume is) a preview of what I'll go through again in my future. I had hot flashes, would sweat even if I wasn't hot, and mood swings. This was on top of everything the chemotherapies were doing to my body concurrently, so it's difficult to isolate exactly what was caused by any single source. But I definitely know that the hot flashes were because of the mini menopause.

When bleeding was no longer as big a concern toward the end of treatment, we stopped the Depo. It took a few months for my cycle to start again and return to normal. *Yay* … the cramps came back full force.

After this long without my normal cycle, the risk of low bone density was a concern. Osteoporosis can happen to anyone, but estrogen is key in retaining calcium. This is why postmenopausal people are more at risk of bone fracture and the like. After I was off the Depo, I had a bone density scan. Thankfully, the results were fine, and I have not come across any late effects (at the moment) as a result of the birth control.

Another outward sign of everything my body was going through—one I couldn't hide—was the hair loss. Strand by strand, my hair fell out. Watching my hair fall out was heartbreaking—not just because I loved my hair, but because it made my illness visible in a way I couldn't control. When I brushed my hair, more fell out. When I would lift my head from my pillow, there would be a shadow of hair where my head had rested. When I touched my scalp, strands would come out in my fingers.

I don't think going bald is easy on anyone. This was emotionally challenging for me, because this was a visual reminder (not that I needed one) that I was sick. Very sick. Everyone around me kept saying not to worry because it would grow back in a few months. But that's not what mattered. I wanted to keep my hair. Who wouldn't? Especially a teenage girl.

When I was diagnosed, I decided I would cut my hair to donate to children who needed wigs since I was going to lose it anyway … and apparently I was going to be one of those kids who would be needing a wig all of a sudden. It actually was the second time I had donated my hair, and I did it again once it came back. A few of my friends went with me to the hairdresser for emotional support. When I saw my short hairdo, I cried. Not because I looked bad. But it was one of those moments when I realized it was going to be a long time before I ever had my own long hair again … if I *ever* had long hair again.

I had this crazy idea that maybe I wouldn't lose *all* my hair. (Denial might be a running theme in my journey.) My doctor had said it was possible it wouldn't all fall out in the first rounds of treatment. So … that could be me. I was fortunate that I never entirely lost my eyelashes or eyebrows; they thinned, but those held on. Apparently brunette hair is "stronger" than other colors and is more likely to make it through chemotherapy.

I did get to the point with my hair that I wanted to shave the rest of it. It was just a few strands, and I thought it would be easier to cope if it was all gone. My parents were nervous about shaving my head because if I got cut, the potential infection could have been horrible with my blood counts. They also had never shaved someone's head before, and I can only assume that allowing me to shave my own head (their child's—little girl's—head) would have been a traumatic experience for them. Anyway, we cut it, but kept the "peach fuzz" that was left behind. Instead of being shiny bald, I looked like the scary decapitated doll/spider creature from *Toy Story*. Adult cancer patients always seem to be beautiful, and kids always seem to be cute (in an extreme, heartbreaking way) when they're bald. I was an ugly bald. (I cry every single time I see a bald child, maybe because I hate to think that they are facing anything like I did. Or that their parents might lose them. That they might not get to grow up or have a normal childhood.)

Every time I saw myself in the mirror from that moment on, I didn't recognize myself. It was as if I thought I would look different, and then this horribly sick girl, a shadow of who I had been, was gawking back at me. I avoided looking in the mirror whenever possible.

When my hair finally did grow back, it came in black and curly. They call that "chemo curls." Your body is so full of the toxins and poisons of chemotherapy that your hair comes out differently and curly. Some people's hair is permanently different, and others go back to normal once the chemo is out of their bodies. My hair started to turn back to its usual brown and straight-as-a-pin about a year later. When my hair was short, I was mistaken for a boy … frequently. If I ever needed an example of why pronouns are important, and you should use a person's chosen pronouns just as you use their chosen name … this was it.

Of course, hair loss was just one sign of the internal warfare my body was enduring. Some of the worst parts weren't visible at all. One of the first chemotherapies I required was on day six in the hospital. It was an intramuscular injection, which the doctors and nurses referred to as "PEG." If you are unfamiliar with intramuscular injections, these have to be administered into your muscles. This one was thrust quickly and deeply into my thigh muscles. This is significantly more agonizing compared to a typical shot that doesn't go into your muscle, but your fat. Once the needles were in the muscle, the chemo itself was far from pleasant. It felt like fire was being inserted into my leg and slowly spread out underneath my skin until it dissipated. Based on my body mass, I had to receive three injections simultaneously to prevent me from having to endure the experience separate times. Before the first time I was going to get the PEGs, they warned me it was not going to be fun. The three nurses surrounded me on the examination table: two on my left, and one on my right (one of my favorite nurses at the time). They counted down, then jabbed. I felt the two go into my left. It was what I would imagine it would feel like to be stabbed with a small knife … two of them. Then the fiery chemo spread into my leg, and it was done. But I didn't feel the one on the right at all. At the time, I thought it was because my favorite nurse did it, and she was just that good. Later, I learned it was something else entirely.

It took a little while before I realized I still wasn't feeling anything on the top of my right leg. Not my pajama pants, nor my hand if I touched it … But occasionally, I was getting the sensation that that part of the leg was asleep. I asked my doctor about why I wasn't feeling normally in that leg. He came, broke a wood splint, and poked around on my leg to see where I could and couldn't feel. He concluded that I must have nerve damage. When he located the least sensitive area, we could see the mark … aka bruise … from the PEG. The injection hit a nerve when it went into my leg, which is why I didn't feel it. He told me the nerve damage was probably permanent, as nerves do not typically regenerate. Needless to say, I was nervous every time I needed the remaining PEG doses.

Over time, the sensation of being asleep, complete with sharp "pins and needles," like the leg was trying to wake up, was a frequent occurrence. And even with the lower regular sensitivity, I was starting to get pain whenever that area was touched. So, if something was on my lap, my right leg would scream until I shifted it to my left.

After treatment, I started to regain some normal feeling in my leg, and the other sensations became fewer and farther between. I'm very glad I have regained the level of normalcy that I have, considering I was told my leg would never recover. Is it perfect? No. Is it way better than when the PEG happened? Absolutely. Still, physical side effects weren't the only thing I had to recover from—there was a lot more going on emotionally, too.

Emotionally, I was unraveling just as my body was trying to stitch itself back together. While each person has a different experience with cancer, it is safe to say that most have a rather difficult time with the adjustments they have to make to their life. Even just the interruptions to your plans … suck. I was *not* one who handled the bulk of my journey with grace. (I am still skeptical that more than a rare few ever are this type but am so proud of anyone who is; they are a million times stronger than I ever will be. I wear my emotions on my sleeves.) I tried as hard and as long as I could to put on a "happy face," but the battles I was fighting inside of my own body were too taxing to be able to keep all my emotions at bay 24/7. Not to mention, some of the medicines I was on had the side effect of mood swings. That *really* didn't help. Between the medications and sheer mental exhaustion, my emotions were constantly in flux. I had moments where I cried frequently, others where I would be upset for no reason, and sometimes I would be fine. I certainly wasn't the most cheerful person to be around.

Looking back, I wish I had been easier on myself—and on those around me. If you're going through cancer treatment, know that it's okay to not feel like yourself. It's okay to be angry or emotional. I would recommend communicating with your support circle so they can understand as best as they can what you're going through (and not to take anything personally). Just remember, that you always know how you're feeling and what is going on in your head. Other people only know what they observe or is told to them. Keep your people in the loop.

If you are caring for someone who is experiencing mood swings or changes that don't seem to be quite them, try not to take it personally. Let them know how you feel and that you are there for them. Take breaks when you need them, and don't forget to take care of yourself as well.

The emotional toll wasn't helped by the fact that what I was going through was written all over my body. Sure, you have good days, when you *could* put makeup and a wig on, but this was **never** who I was. Getting "pretty" was never something I did for myself when I had energy and was healthy. So feeling as if I was being forced to do it when I was fatigued and felt like the walking dead was for other people's sake, not mine. Doing your hair and makeup takes *time* and *energy*. You have a finite amount of both. How you decide to use them is up to you. On good days, I wanted to savor each moment instead of wasting it doing a routine I loathed. And on bad days? You get what you get with me. That is always how I have been, and I was not going to let cancer change that. There was enough it was taking from me. It was not going to change the essence of who I was. (There *is* more to me than being stubborn, but I hope you know what I mean.)

Adding to the many physical tolls, lumbar punctures—or "LPs"—were a regular part of treatment throughout most phases. For these, unlike the very first one done while my port was being placed, they would be done in a special room in the clinic. (One was done in my hospital room, and they later had to occur in the radiology department.) The room had a flat table, on which you had to remain an hour after the puncture (to rebalance your equilibrium because your spinal fluid had been thrown off, resulting in killer headaches). During these, the same thing would happen like the first time: a sample of my spinal fluid would be taken to be tested, and intrathecal methotrexate would be injected. Sometimes, I would also have a bone marrow aspirate. These were only to test the bone marrow, so was not done as often as the LPs. I did ask to see my bone marrow and spinal fluid once … Because, *why not?* How many people have seen their own marrow and spinal fluid?

During the LP and aspiration procedures, I would be hooked up to an oxygen sensor and heart monitor and given "conscious sedation." The conscious sedation would make me forget most of the experience and would make me loopy (I assumed this would be similar to when people get their wisdom teeth removed, and others occasionally film how they act when they're high), but otherwise I was *technically* conscious. My family never filmed me … but they should have. I came up with what I thought were the best ideas after these procedures while I was under the influence of the medicines. And the way in which I delivered the ideas, I'm told, was quite humorous.

One of the first million-dollar ideas while high was around Christmas time. After the procedure, my family took me down to the cafeteria in a wheelchair (since I was still loopy) to see the gingerbread houses that had been built (by whom, I have no idea). You could smell the sugar before even getting off the elevator. Looking at the houses, I had the brilliant idea (and I still stand by this) that instead of gingerbread, you should build houses out of Rice Krispies Treats. This could be done in two ways: make the walls as one giant treat, and glue them together with frosting, or build your house out of smaller treats like bricks. Gingerbread is not easy to stick together. (My brother and I struggled with that each year at the teen group Christmas party.) But Rice Krispies Treats are quite sticky. And they're already white, so making it look like snow would be easy. And this wasn't just an idea, but one I was trying very hard to sell to my family (as if it were the most important thing I'd ever said in my life). Yeah … D.J. made fun of me for that one. And then Rice Krispies Treats started selling a gingerbread house kit a year or two later! Eventually I started falling asleep during the procedures; there wasn't quite the same aftereffect, and I wasn't as amusing.

Soon, my skin hurt all over as if I had a horrible sunburn. Before the LP needle could be inserted into my back, the doctor had to press around my vertebrae to find the exact spot. Eventually, the pressure from this was more painful than the needle itself. Even with sedation, I would react whenever my back was pushed. One time, I was told later, I reacted before the doctor even touched me. They found it comical that I was more sensitive to the touch of my skin than to the needle itself. As for what I did while unconscious? I'm not responsible—I just remember how much my skin *hurt*.

One day when I went in for the LP, the oxygen sensor seemed to be malfunctioning. I distinctly remember wondering, *"Is that really necessary for such a routine procedure?"* But then I thought, *"What if I need it today of all days?"* When I went under, I apparently slipped into sedation too quickly. The next thing I remember is waking up surrounded by more people than should have been there.

Something was wrong.

I also felt something odd, like something was inside my back … *Yup, that was a long needle in there. Were they doing the LP **right now**?* I was more lucid than normal at this point of becoming conscious and quite aware of my surroundings.

My mom looked really nervous. She had that look of worry on her face only a parent can have over their child.

Like I had just done something that she never wanted me to do again.

And everything else I know from that point forward is from my mom and my doctor's recount of events.

I had stopped breathing right at the beginning of the procedure. How often have we checked for the gentle rise and fall of one of our loved one's chests as they slumber, even though a part of us knows … *assumes* … of course they are still breathing? Why on earth would they not be?

My mom noticed I had stopped breathing. My doctor didn't seem to believe her at first, because the medications can slow your breathing … but this time, mine slowed until it stopped altogether. My brain had ceased to remind my body to keep itself alive with one of the basic functions it normally does autonomously (which is terrifying it can do that). They had to call a code, and everyone … *everyone* … rushed into the room to resuscitate me. They reversed the sedation medication and thankfully got me to start breathing on my own. When I was breathing again, my doctor decided to do the LP before everything fully wore off so he wouldn't have to try again the next day (since it's not possible to sedate you twice like that, especially after a reaction like I had).

This was a jarring moment—it left me with a heavy load of trauma. The reality hit me hard: I could have easily died without waking up. It didn't make sense—what a strange way to go, for my own brain to forget to keep me alive. Besides, there was so much more I wanted to do. I hadn't even met Johnny Depp yet, and I really wanted to act alongside him. *A girl can dream, right?*

When all was said and done, I asked my mom to take me to school, even though the day was over. I had to talk to my Chemistry teacher for some reason. Life was too precious to wait.

When I got to school, it was really sinking in how close I came to losing my life that day. Walking down the hallways I had walked a million times, that day felt different. I unloaded *a lot* on my teacher, and we had a really heavy conversation. (If you ever read this, I'm so sorry … but thank you.)

After a few more LPs, the low vertebrae that my oncologist used to access became entirely blocked by scar tissue, which made it impenetrable. When I woke from one LP attempt and asked how it went, my doctor said he couldn't do it. That's when he explained I would return the next day so he could try again. Without being able to access that area, that meant they had to move up another vertebra higher on my back. The higher up on the backbone you move, the greater the risk of hitting the spinal cord or a nerve. This risk meant that before the needle could go in, they had to make sure nothing (like the spinal cord) was in the way. This required going to the radiology department, and they would use a machine to see my spinal column before accessing me. Only an oncologist could administer the methotrexate (or any chemotherapy), so my doctor would come down to the radiology department once I was accessed and ready for the medicine to be given. I'm grateful for the talented doctors and equipment they used and that everything else went smoothly.

It might be safe to say—though I acknowledge it could have been far worse—that lumbar punctures left their mark on me. Not just physically, but emotionally. I don't know how much I processed the gravity of how close I came to dying on the table. If my mom had not spoken up immediately when I stopped breathing, who knows how long it might have taken for someone else to notice.

Did you know at three minutes without oxygen, lasting brain damage is likely? After ten minutes without breathing, you are unlikely to recover? An LP takes on average between fifteen and thirty minutes. I was extremely lucky. But I could have just as easily not been lucky.

I try not to dwell on situations like this. In fact, the way I tend to deal with them is to either subconsciously block it out or actively try to not think about it at all. So … I don't really deal with them at all. I realize that isn't the healthiest way to cope, but I try to stay positive (and negative experiences can be difficult to process). I realize now how beneficial it would have been to go to therapy during treatment.

For the longest time, hearing the letters "LP" felt like being hit by a wave I never saw coming—a tsunami of memories, fear, and pain that I wasn't ready to confront. It was, without question, a trigger. In my brain, "LP" was synonymous with *lumbar puncture*. The emotional aftermath of what happened during that LP haunted me for years. The mere mention of those two letters could send my heart racing and my mind spiraling back to a place I would rather have left behind.

Writing this memoir has helped me begin to unpack the weight of those associations—peeling back the layers of fear, anger, and helplessness I buried deep in the moment just to survive. But healing doesn't always arrive in the ways we expect. Sometimes, it shows up quietly, wrapped beautifully in something entirely different. For me, that unexpected balm came in the form of my favorite actress—Lana Parrilla—probably best known for her role as the Evil Queen in *Once Upon a Time*. She's often referred to as "LP."

Once Upon a Time aired after my active treatment ended, but it entered my life when I still desperately needed stories of resilience, second chances, and the possibility of a happy ending. Watching the show (and everything else Lana has been in) on what could only be described as an endless loop gave me something to hold on to—something joyful, powerful, and hopeful. Over time, those two letters—LP—stopped pulling me back into trauma and started leading me toward comfort, creativity, and connection. Now, when I hear them, I think not of pain, but of someone whose work helped me find light in the shadows.

You may have noticed a pattern: I love deeply, and I tend to find extraordinary joy in the artists I admire. Lana Parrilla, "LP," became more than a distraction—she became a part of my healing. And in that unexpected turn, I found yet another piece of myself (along with several new friends in the "Evil Regal" community).

While healing emotionally was one part of the journey, (and has taken years after treatment to get where I am today) the physical environment of the hospital constantly reminded me of the reality I was living. The routines, the smells, and the isolation all became a backdrop to my experience.

When you are in the hospital, everyone "scrubs in and out" when they come into your room. There are Purell dispensers on the walls next to every room's doorway which provide a quick squirt of the hand sanitizer. You get used to that smell. Everyone who comes near you has the sweet, tangy smell of the quick evaporating gel. I'm honestly surprised that smell doesn't bother me today because of how often it was ever-present. Occasionally, I would win an isolation experience (as if having cancer and being in the hospital wasn't enough of an isolating experience).

Isolation would involve an extra few steps to enter the room. You had to wear a mask (before that was a thing common people did), dress in a hospital gown, and wash your hands with warm water and soap. Instant hand sanitizer wasn't enough. It may kill 99.99% of germs, but whatever is going on to put you in isolation falls into that 0.01%. Sometimes the isolation was to protect you (like if your counts were so low that the most innocent microbe could take you down), and other times, you were the danger.

There was one hospital stay they didn't know what was wrong with me. (That seemed to be a recurring theme with me; I'm not sure if being unique with your medical journey is a good thing.) Whatever I may have had could have been one of those 0.01% of bacteria that only real old-school hand-washing could take care of.

This was one of the pleasant times I needed to have a commode in my room. This was a low point in my journey, and I may very well cut this part out of the final memoir and am 100% not even writing about something else that happened. (I guess you'll just have to use your imagination on that one … or don't … please don't.) If you do not know what a commode is, it's a portable toilet. I had a private bathroom in my hospital room, but there were a few times in my treatment that I was not able to make it the few feet from my hospital bed to the bathroom. This particular time I was in isolation was one of those where I had very little control over my body. I felt as if I went from being a teenager, and pediatric, directly to being geriatric. It was embarrassing (but could have been worse), but you do what you have to do and keep moving forward (even though I felt as if I was moving backward as I was losing the ability to do basic functions).

While they were trying to figure out what was wrong, they made me stop eating for a few days. (That's one of the cruelest forms of punishment for me.) They thought I could have had a reaction in my body that would have been dangerous for anything to be inside my intestinal tract as it would have become damaged and infected if it was inflamed. It thankfully began to get better in a few more days and I was allowed to eat again.

The first year of treatment was cycling between being in the hospital and then home. When I was home, I spent most of my days on the couch, watching entire series of TV shows because I was too fatigued to do much. While I was in the hospital (wishing I was home), I "slept" to Nick at Night (a late hour takeover of the Nickelodeon channel).

I'm not going to lie, being able to watch TV late at night when I should have been asleep was pretty cool. In my house, you did not have a TV in your bedroom. I'll never forget waking up a few times in the middle of the night when I was young and seeing that the family room TV was on. The light from the screen would flicker against the hallway wall, and the soft volume could just be made out if you stretched to listen for it. That meant that one of my parents was awake, and maybe they would let me come and watch with them. For some reason, the same thing you would do during the day was a million times more fun at night when you were supposed to be in bed. So when I had a TV in my hospital room and trouble sleeping (my whole schedule was off once I began treatment), watching shows in the middle of the night was sort of cool.

But while late-night TV offered a small comfort during those sleepless nights, the reality of treatment was never far away. The first—and most intense—phase was called "induction," where the doctors aimed to get me into remission with a powerful cocktail of chemotherapies. But just because you enter remission doesn't mean that you're out of the woods. There are still lingering leukemia cells that cannot be detected. So, on to the next rounds.

The names of the next few rounds until the final are a little blurry. I remember the words "intensification," "consolidation," and "delayed intensification." What order they came in, how long they lasted, and the exact nuances of how they differed, I can no longer put my finger on. I vaguely remember something also having a "2," like a sequel … but I could entirely be making that up.

Depending on the phase, there were different chemo combinations and requirements. One required outpatient infusions that lasted a few hours. This meant I would go to the hospital, get hooked up to machines as if I was admitted, but get to leave at the end of the day. A different phase required inpatient infusions, where I was checked in for a few days (or more). It was methotrexate in a lime-green solution, which would take 24 hours to get into me. Afterward, they had to flush it out of my system, so I would be in the hospital a few more days having fluid pumped quickly through me (and peeing … *lots* of peeing). These weeks were "fun," because this is when I would get horrible blister-like mouth sores. While I had these, nothing could go into my mouth without causing excruciating pain. I'm grateful for the miracle mouthwash that made eating and drinking *almost* possible (as it would numb my mouth for a few minutes … and everything tasted like mint because of the medicine).

Eventually, we figured out a small reason I was getting such severe side effects was because I was deficient in an enzyme in my body that helps to break down some of the chemotherapies. So the medicines were staying in my system longer than they should have, which was the equivalent of receiving a higher dose than the doctors counted on. Going forward after this discovery, some doses had to be adjusted to compensate. One of which was the intravenous methotrexate. They reduced the dilution by 25%, and it was a lighter green the next time around. Still the same amount of fluid and theoretically the medicine would be in my system the same amount of time as 100% should have been.

The next time after that, the bag of methotrexate was not the same light green I was expecting … it was even lighter. I questioned why it wasn't the same color and was told it had been reduced by 25%. I asked why that had been done a second time, which took the person administering it aback. They had to go and ask. When they returned, there had been a mistake while reading my chart, as it was supposed to be the same as the previous time. Since this bag was already made up, they made another bag to get the rest of the medicine in without wasting the one that was ready. So I had the pleasure of having twice as much fluid pumped through me that day. (They had to compensate for twice the fluid by increasing the speed it would go into me.) I should have just stayed in the bathroom that day, since I kept turning back around to pee again. (The lesson here? Learn your chemistry dilutions and concentration calculations if you're interested in going into the medical field. And always ask questions when you don't think something is right.)

Alongside the challenges of methotrexate, another medication I struggled with was the steroid prednisone—one that brought its own set of difficult side effects. I hated that medicine. (Most were unpleasant, but this one struck a nerve … not in the same way the PEGs did.) During one phase, I would be on it for several days and then stop taking it, which would cause me to get migraines. If you have never had the pleasure of experiencing a migraine, it can range from person to person.

I can explain mine.

It starts with an aura in my field of vision. The aura appears to be sparkly lights that grow and slowly take over my eyesight (even when my eyes are closed). Then comes the pain. My head feels as if it is being squeezed in a table vise and scooped out by a melon baller. Light and sound *hurt*. Nausea overcomes me. And the only thing I can do to find some relief is to fall asleep in a quiet, dark room. When I wake up, it is either gone (hopefully) or a dull but tolerable-in-comparison throbbing remains. Acetaminophen helps a little, but once one starts, it's too late. One benefit to cancer treatment was we discovered a preventative medicine that still keeps most of my migraines at bay. Unfortunately, as I look ahead at wanting to start a family (assuming that's medically possible), I will have to come off this medicine.

Despite these tough side effects, the bigger battle was always keeping my blood counts high enough to continue treatment. There were one or two times I was supposed to start the next round of chemo, but my blood counts were too low. I remember one semi-vividly. My mom said she had to tell me something. (I thought she was going to tell me I had relapsed.) It was in her pre-K classroom after the school day.

My mom taught preschool for most of my life, and my family would often help her bring her supplies into the room to set up for the day or pick everything up. She did so many creative projects and lessons that required prep work at home.

My mom sat me down at one of the tiny tables built for the three-year-olds. She said the doctors didn't find any cell growth in my bone marrow when they tested it.

I took that as a good sign. If even all the healthy cells were wiped out, clearly the cancer cells had to be, too. It took a while for my counts to bounce back so I could move on to the next treatment phase. But I was optimistic from that point about my prognosis.

From the moment I started treatment, I did what I had to do. My entire family did. What was the alternative? The goal was to get to the final round, "maintenance." That was when the intensity of the chemo lightened, and I would begin to regain some sense of normalcy. This was when I was told my hair would start growing back (which it did). It was a sign I would almost be at the end of the tunnel. That doesn't mean it was all sunshine and flowers. But it was a monumental step in the right direction.

Before reaching the relative relief of maintenance, though, I had to survive what would become my darkest hour. Of everything I'd dealt with, my rock bottom was something that likely could have been handled a little differently. I had been in the hospital for a few weeks, on the highest amount of painkillers I was able to have because I was quite sick and in severe pain. Morphine didn't seem to have any effect on me, so stronger medicines were used. There is a difference between *pain* and *discomfort*, which you learn when you're going through something as strenuous as cancer treatment. Something can be *unpleasant* without being *painful*. Those few weeks, I was in *pain*. The amount of drugs I was given kept me in a constant cycle of semi-conscious, unconscious moments. I would see that someone had come to visit, close my eyes, and open them the next day. Or my family would put a movie on, I'd blink, and the end credits would be rolling. Even at these points, it is humbling to remember that someone is always facing something worse than you are. Even at my low points, I had a lot to be grateful for.

When I came out of whatever it was that was keeping me down, I was taken straight off the painkillers and sent home. And I immediately felt … off.

At the time, we didn't know what was happening to me. Later on, we realized the horrible experience I went through was withdrawal. If I had ever needed more reason to not abuse medication (I didn't need *any* more reasons, and even was resistant to using the medication when it was absolutely necessary), this was it. I'm not going to dwell on this for too long … But it sucked. If this is a trigger warning for you, maybe skip to the next section.

I spent most of my time over the next few days on the loveseat in our family room, where I could watch TV. At first, I started to lose every liquid from inside my body. However it could come out, it did. I could not eat. (Which on its own is a horrendous effect, as food is *amazing*.) I was hot and cold at the same time, sweating profusely and shivering simultaneously. My body ached, and my legs were restless. My shins burned like they wanted to get up and move, but I didn't have the energy to. At least sleep should have been a respite … but it would not come.

The first twenty-four hours were bad, but we have all been ill for that long before, so it wasn't the end of the world. Surely sleep was around the corner.

Again, I could not sleep the second evening.

On the third, I took one of my sleeping pills. I didn't like to do this because they had given me extremely vivid nightmares when I took them at the beginning of treatment. But after three days of withdrawal and not sleeping, I was willing to take sleep with nightmares over no sleep.

I still didn't sleep that third evening and was beginning to lose my mind. On top of feeling like utter crap, I was beyond exhausted. I had always enjoyed sleeping, and this was getting old … fast.

I tried another sleeping pill on the fourth evening. This *had* to be the night. You can't stay awake forever. The longest on record seems to be eleven days, but who the heck would want to be awake for that long?! Unfortunately, I'm not exaggerating how long I went without sleep, as this is not something I'm proud of one iota. The medicine would surely help me fall asleep for at least a little while.

That evening is when it got dark. (Every evening is *dark*, but my mind went to a dark place.) I am not proud of any thoughts I had, but I didn't seriously take them anywhere.

In the middle of that fourth sleepless night, where I was still expelling the toxins from my body in the most unpleasant ways possible and begging for shuteye, I came to the realization that this was not sustainable. I could not live like this for long. Living without sleep alone, perfectly healthy otherwise, could not be done indefinitely. If I didn't find sleep or otherwise get better soon, I would not be able to keep going. This almost broke me to a point I didn't think I'd come back from. This could have been the end of my journey.

But I had a voice in the back of my head that said I had to find a way to keep going, to keep holding on. *Pirates of the Caribbean 4* had not come out yet, and I still had to meet (and act with) Johnny Depp. There was too much to live for … to keep fighting for.

On the fifth day, I started to feel a little more stable (less "leaky"), and finally (*for the love of God*) fell asleep that evening. Even if it wasn't the best night's sleep ever, it was extremely welcomed and gave promise of the future.

I wouldn't wish what I went through those days on my worst enemy. And if you're ever in a dark place, there are people who care and can help. At the very least, just a phone call away.

Once I clawed my way out of that physical and emotional mess, I figured things could only get better. And they did—sort of. I wasn't in such a dark place anymore.

Think of your most embarrassing memory. I'll give you a minute … Do you have one in mind? You don't have to tell anyone what it is (unless you laugh about it now). Now let me tell you about one of my most embarrassing moments, and hopefully you'll feel a tad better about your own. Or perhaps I'm being overly dramatic about mine, and you should share yours with me some day.

When you're on a cocktail of medications that can dry out your whole system (for example … chemo), it's perfectly reasonable that your doctors might be concerned that you will become constipated (which isn't pleasant when you are healthy and comfortable). Now … perhaps TMI (I would assume this whole book is a bit too much info) … I was *regular*, but not *daily* regular. Well, they wanted me *daily* regular and were going to check up on that … at the most inopportune times.

I was eating? *Perfect.* I had company? *Even better.*

If the doctors had a discreet code, like "everything come out okay?", maybe that wouldn't have been so bad. But no. They always wanted to know details.

"Have you had a bowel movement today? You haven't? Have you tried yet? Does it hurt when you push? Have you taken your laxatives? I'll get you more." Because laxatives were part of the regimen.

I think it was even worse if it *had* happened before the doctor made their rounds.

"Can you describe the consistency for me? What color was it? Anything else of note?"

Like, *holy crap* (literally). I really didn't want my friends or other visitors to hear all of that. Even alone, that's weird to talk to another person about.

What was even a step worse than that was when I had a skin reaction in a very inconvenient location … I don't even want to type this … Let's just say that it was on the right side of the very top of my left leg … Okay, it was on my butt, but not quite visible from afar … I'll spare you the worst of the mental imagery, but just know: it was not glamorous, and it definitely wasn't getting better. It was em-bare-assing (pun intended) enough just having the abrasion, let alone having to tell my doctor about it (because it was concerning that it wasn't healing). Of course, that meant they had to look. Once … whatever. I had little shame at that point. But since it wasn't healing, and a risk for infection, they had to keep looking at it a few times a day.

Several times, the doctor wasn't alone. It was common at my hospital for there to be doctors or nurses in training that would accompany the other medical professionals on rounds so they could gain experience and learn. I'm sure this wasn't the worst thing they had to see, but it felt like it to me.

This was also one of those rounds where it didn't matter if you had company … "Can we look at it?" Of course there were privacy curtains and people in my room would leave, but that is super awkward for a teenager. *Hey guys, can these people just look at my butt, then we can get back to the game we were playing?* Don't get me wrong. I know the doctors were just doing their job (and did an incredible job that saved my life). I'd assume that they were just on a tight schedule with everything they had to do and were desensitized to certain things.

So … How did I do? If your story wins, you must find me and share it with me one day. If you're laughing at me, that's okay. I've gotten to that point myself.

After all that awkwardness, it was a relief to find joy in the small things—and one of those small but meaningful joys was food. Not just eating, but the little rituals around it that made me feel a bit more like myself. Sometimes I got to go to the cafeteria with a voucher, in place of having a meal delivered to my room, and pick out whatever I wanted (like a normal visitor or outpatient person could do). It just tasted better from there. Maybe because it wasn't steamed under the aquamarine Tupperware cloche used to keep the meals warm on their delivery. It was also like a mini field trip, even if I was only getting off MS8 for a few minutes. I did have to be supervised, and it was more fun when I went down with my family (but some great people on staff sometimes took me).

The snacks I was able to get in the cafeteria, but not off the menu, were great. There were fun ice creams, dessert parfaits, soft pretzels, popcorn, cheesecake, soup, pizza (you know, super nutritional stuff) … *Yum.*

When I did order off the menu, I had to order the day before (or request the voucher). There were some things that were always available (like hamburgers, hot dogs, chicken tenders). But for each day of the week, there were specials in addition to the usual menu. There were a few that I liked, and I would wait all week for them. Until someone mentioned to us that we could request the specials on any day. The cafeteria workers were great and let me do just that. For a while, all I ate were the tacos until medically they wouldn't let me eat the chicken because it could have interacted with my medicines. Then I ate the mini pot pies … Until *Sweeney Todd* ruined that for me.

I didn't have as much of an appetite as I normally did. (Nausea is a huge side effect of chemo; thankfully I didn't throw up frequently.) So when I was in the mood for something, my family was wonderful and helped me get it. Food has always been a comfort for me. I am one of those people who live to eat (as opposed to eating to live). I ate bags of lightly salted potato chips. My brother and dad would get kid's meals from the Friendly's next door to the hospital. There was a triple chocolate muffin at the Dunkin across the street for a few weeks. My uncle and aunt brought up my favorite mac and cheese from Outback one time. When we were out of the hospital, as much as I still liked food, I could not eat an adult-sized meal. (I was still a teenager and quite short, so even without being sick, my stomach was not very spacious, although it was padded.) I remember being turned down for a kid's meal, even though I was still young, and you could tell I was sick. Granted, the age limit was a few years below me. But I wasn't trying to get anything special, just a smaller-sized portion (which I think every restaurant should offer the option of smaller portions for all ages).

I had a "food bucket list" for when I was feeling well enough and out of the hospital, that I wanted to eat (morbidly, *at least one last time*). I still have that list. There are so many things on it that have since been discontinued, but I got almost all of them while I was sick. My mom and I would get original recipe chicken wings from KFC frequently because we both liked those. My family even brought me my favorite pizza from the shore area (about an hour away) once. Unfortunately, I was never able to eat it because I was not feeling great at the time. But it's the thought that counts, and I will always remember that they went out of their way to bring it to me, and the lovely note that was written in one of the boxes by our favorite server. (Who we bonded with after learning she lost a daughter to cancer … It's crazy how something as horrible as cancer can bond you instantly with others.)

Still, even with all that effort to chase cravings and check off items from my food bucket list, my appetite wasn't always consistent. Over time, the doctors got worried I wasn't eating enough (I thought I was), so they gave me snacks every few hours in between meals. I had an additional menu for these, which had really cool things like *real* milkshakes (as opposed to the packaged ones that tasted like milk with the calories of a milkshake) and cans of Pringles.

At the beginning of treatment, I really liked the chicken tenders offered in the cafeteria. These were one of the only things that were good steamed from the plastic cloche you would get inpatient, or the Styrofoam box while outpatient (as you could get lunches if you were in the clinic all day), or directly from the cafeteria. (The hamburger was also good but tasted super different depending which way you got it. I think more spices were added to the "general public" food.) But one day while I was in the clinic eating lunch, staring at the tenders in their white Styrofoam box, it hit me … *I'll be eating this for several meals over the next 2 plus years.* That felt like an eternity I didn't even know would come to an end, and I couldn't stomach even the smell anymore. It was an immediate gag reflex check each time I smelled them. (Chemo made some smells repulsive, even if they had never bothered me before.) I felt bad, because the smell would turn my stomach from that point, so I didn't even want my family to order it.

Chemotherapy is known for several things, one of which is making the patient nauseated. I don't think I have ever met someone who enjoys tossing their cookies, but I hate it on a different level. I dislike it so much that my brain usually overpowers my natural instincts to throw up. When I realized I was likely going to be nauseous constantly, I was not excited (Again, who would be?). Thankfully, there was an anti-nausea medication to help with the sensation, which did help. I probably threw up less than ten times over the two and a half years.

But there was one medicine in particular that betrayed me … I would take it, and everything would immediately come back up. Even if I tried covering my nose so I wouldn't taste it (I think it was bubble gum flavored or something gross), I would immediately eject everything. It's almost as if I was allergic to the texture (it felt like sand in milk), if that was even possible. After a few times, I stopped taking it altogether. It was supposed to coat the digestive track before eating to protect it from potential scrapes or tears. But I would rather risk putting food in my untreated system than whatever damage tossing my cookies was doing.

But there were many more changes, in addition to nausea, that chemo brought. When you are experiencing something traumatic, such as intensive chemotherapy (or surgery or radiation), your body goes through a lot of changes. Some are temporary, and some may be permanent. As I progressed through the rounds of chemo, I saw different aspects of my abilities regress. It can be difficult for anyone to watch themselves physically deteriorate in any respect. At sixteen, I had not considered that I would be in that boat of watching my body fail at what I wanted it to do. It was emotionally challenging to see what I could no longer do and didn't know if I ever would be able to again.

At first, I saw my handwriting get messier because my hands were sore and no longer had the strength to hold a writing utensil the way they used to.

Next (because of the same medicine that took my neat and pain-free handwriting—Vincristine), my legs became limited in their abilities. Now, I am extremely grateful I was always able to walk. I know that there was always a miniscule risk with each lumbar puncture that I could have forever lost that ability in a split second. And obviously if my situation was any different, I could have lost that ability temporarily or permanently for other reasons. But that doesn't mean it wasn't still emotionally difficult to cope with the limitations I had.

I developed "foot drop." When you walk normally, your heel hits the ground first, then you sort of roll it and move onto the ball of your foot before lifting your heel and foot at the end of your step. Foot drop is when you can't lift the front part of your foot. So when you walk, your heel hits the ground, and instead of rolling, your whole foot essentially slaps down. I no longer had the capacity to stand on my heels if I wanted to because the muscles simply would not work that way anymore. I could stand on my toes if I wanted, and it actually became easier to walk that way versus slapping around all the time.

This helped make it so I was unable to run (not that I was going to be doing any marathons … ever), but I was incapable of moving any quicker than a slow walk because my legs would give out if my brain tried to have them move any faster than that.

Because of this, I was also unable to walk up or down stairs. My legs did not have the strength to lift me up from one step to the next, nor were they reliable enough to catch me stepping down. If you are fully capable of walking flights of stairs, you might not think about how prevalent they are … they are EVERYWHERE. More places need to be handicap accessible.

I had physical therapy to try to help with stairs. They would take me (with my walker … yup, I needed a walker) to the stairs between MS8 and the seventh floor and try to help me work on going up or down. It didn't really work. As long as I was going to be on the medicine that was doing this to my legs, I was going to struggle with these issues.

Because walking was such a challenge, the medical personnel wanted me to use a walker. It had more support than a cane, but it felt too much in the way for me. I felt myself bending over it more than I should have, which also became a fall risk. I asked to use a cane instead, but for some reason that didn't go anywhere. In the end (and the therapy helped a bit), I was in an okay enough position that I didn't have to use the walker once I left the hospital. Although, having a cane would have been helpful at times.

A while after the leg weakness began, my shoulders began to fail. They became excruciatingly agonizing (as if they were shattered), and I could no longer lift my arms over my head. If anyone tries to tell you bones can't hurt, they're wrong. I had never realized how much I had become dependent on the ability to lift my arms over my head (or have a decent range of motion with them, period). I was planning to become a teacher. In that state, there was no way I would be able to write on a whiteboard if I could only lift my arms as high as my face (especially as I'm short). I couldn't shave under my arms (gross, but necessary). And possibly the worst? I would get trapped in clothes. Some shirts would go on easily, but then I couldn't get them off. They would slide right over my shoulders and arms like the head of an arrow or harpoon. But when I would go to take them off, since my arms couldn't move very much, the shirts would get stuck underneath, and I was not able to wiggle my way out. That seems silly, but I had a few close calls when I was alone (in a dressing room or just in general when I was changing) that I didn't even have anyone I could ask for help if I couldn't figure it out myself. I realized that I could not be as independent as I wanted to be, and sometimes had to ask someone to help me undress when all else failed.

As much as my shoulders physically hurt (a constant and intense burning pain from the inside), the limited range of motion was just as painful. This caused me to search for an answer and possible solution (because living with my shoulders like this forever was not a realistic option I was willing to accept).

The first diagnosis I was given was frozen shoulder (which involves stiffness and pain in your shoulder, which then causes it to become immobile). I even went to physical therapy for a while for this. Everyone kept saying "you're so young for frozen shoulders," and "how strange to get it in both shoulders at once." That should have been a sign, but I had been through so much at that point, my body was acting fifty years older than it actually was. After a while, someone suggested I see an orthopedic specialist and get a second opinion.

They, too, thought it was frozen shoulder at first. They were basically like "why are you here if you already knew that?" But they didn't like that I was so young, so they poked a little deeper. They asked about the medications I was on or had taken. THIS IS A HUGE THING TO KEEP IN MIND IF YOU ARE EVER SEEKING MEDICAL TREATMENT AFTER CANCER CARE! Side effects can happen *way* after you are done taking a medicine like chemotherapy (these are called late effects). The doctors treating you *need* to understand your medical history and hypothetical late effects! When I said the word "prednisone," a lightbulb went off in their head. They pulled my x-rays out and looked again. I don't quite understand why it wasn't able to be seen before (probably because they weren't looking for it), but it was suddenly visible to them.

I had severe avascular necrosis (AVN). The prednisone (a steroid) had cut the blood flow off to my shoulders, and the bones had died. I did not like that diagnosis. My friend had just had a complete knee replacement since she had AVN in her knee. But I asked what I already knew the answer to. *What are my options?* I was told that AVN did not get better. I could either have both shoulders replaced or live with the pain and limited mobility. They suggested a double shoulder replacement and referred me to an orthopedic surgeon.

My mom took me to the orthopedic surgeon, who said the same thing. There were options on the types of shoulders I could get. Some lasted longer than others, but all would almost definitely have to be replaced several times in my lifetime. I did the math in my head. I was about eighteen at the time. I was given an estimate of fifteen years (on the high end) of the life expectancy of the replacement, and each subsequent one would likely last less because of the wear and tear on the joint. *Multiplied by two shoulders … Even if my life expectancy is possibly shorter after everything …* That was *way* more surgery than I was willing to sign up for. Not to mention I was still on my parents' insurance, and I already had the preexisting "cancer" condition. I didn't need to be entirely uninsurable.

I asked basic questions.

Was surgery going to make the pain go away? Most likely.

Was it going to help with my mobility? Maybe.

Um … mobility was a huge deal for me. Before I signed up for potentially three or more double shoulder replacements in my life, I wanted a *guarantee* that I would be able to use my arms as normal again. (Or better! With bionic or whatnot …) They could not give that to me. So, me being the stubborn person that I am, and since shoulders aren't load-bearing joints, I waited. I returned for follow-ups to keep an eye on my shoulders. There was no change the next time or two.

In between, I was weaned off the prednisone because it was damaging my bones. When the damage outweighs the benefits of the medicine, it's not worth continuing. Then, the shoulder pain slowly stopped. I still couldn't really move my arms, but they didn't hurt as much. Baby steps.

At my next checkup, something incredible happened. My surgeon said my x-rays were an improvement from the last ones. There had been bone regeneration! They were shocked; severe AVN tends to be irreversible. But it looked like my shoulders would come back to life. Slowly, I regained range of motion in both shoulders and am near where I was beforehand. My shoulders just get stiff and crack occasionally now and are sometimes sore for no reason. *So* much better considering I didn't go through with the replacements. Will I need surgery one day? Who knows?

While my shoulders were healing, my legs remained weak, sometimes giving out unexpectedly. This led to moments where I literally couldn't get up on my own—which reminded me of those "Help! I've fallen and I can't get up" commercials. Though those advertisements can seem exaggerated, they reflect the real struggles people with invisible disabilities face.

Thankfully, I didn't get seriously injured when I fell. I suppose in a way, it was a blessing that I could not walk up and down stairs at this point, because I most certainly would have taken a nasty tumble with how unpredictable my footing was.

Falling down was bad and embarrassing enough (although, it was even worse when I was alone), but once I was on the ground, I didn't have the upper body strength to get myself back up. (Now, my husband or brother might joke about how I still don't have upper body strength …) My arms were like Harry Potter's when the bones were removed from his arm in the second book/movie after he broke it … They felt like jelly. I would try to push myself up, and nothing would happen.

I deeply understand those commercials now. Falling and not being able to get up is terrifying. I vividly remember falling down once in the movie theater (where my family picked me up), once outside of my house, and once alone in the high school hallway after school. Again, I realized I couldn't be as independent as I wanted, which sucked.

At my house, I went outside before anyone else, and we had one step to get down to the driveway. I stepped down (as carefully as possible because any stair was nearly impossible), and my leg did not support me. I went down and remember thinking I was so glad someone else was going to be coming out soon. I tried to get up, but it was no use. Within a few moments, one of my family members saw I was imitating a welcome mat and helped me up.

At school, it was a different situation. I had gone to visit teachers I hadn't seen since I left in November. It was a little past the time you'd expect every teacher to still be there (because they have lives of their own), but that was the quickest I could get to the school because of coming from the hospital (which always took longer than you thought it would, even if you were fortunate to be only outpatient that day). Plus, it wasn't a great idea to go when there were still students in the building as more people equaled a higher chance of catching something.

I was in a hallway in the back of the school, after I had already said hi to a few teachers (so it was really late at this point). I thought I would try one more teacher before heading out.

The hallway was entirely empty. I could tell the teacher had left, which I expected (but at this point, it wasn't every day I was allowed or able to visit the school, so I wanted to confirm). I also had to walk a certain direction, because one hallway had stairs, and the other had a ramp. I had to take the path with the ramp. I wasn't even walking quickly (not that I could at this point). I just wiped out. Some people have a talent for tripping on air (which I possess), but these falls were more that my legs would become wobbly for a moment and forget how to support me. I'd collapse down onto myself. This time was horrifying because I didn't know how I would get up or when I'd be found. I had no idea when would be the next time someone would walk by. I needed either a person or something like a chair to help pull myself up. Looking around, I was in a slippery hallway with locked doors and lockers out of reach. There was nothing I would be able to use to support myself to get up.

So, this is how I die after everything I've been through.

Okay, I may have been a tad dramatic, but this was scary. This also wasn't a time where everyone had cell phones and I could call for help. I didn't even know if anyone was in the main office and would be able to help locate me on cameras if my ride started to get concerned I wasn't coming out. As embarrassing as falling in front of another would have been, I really wanted someone to be there to help me up … or at least get help.

I tried to push myself off the ground and back onto my feet. Nothing.

My body may have appeared weak and useless, but it was doing a remarkable job on the inside fighting for my life. I really underappreciated its strength because of moments such as this. But after reflecting on all it accomplished and got me through, I realized it's strong in different ways.

I lost track of time. Eventually, a custodian came by. I'm sure that was not what they were expecting to clean off the floor: a sickly girl sprawled on the ground. Even though I had been hoping someone would come by, I was still super embarrassed. All too excitedly, I called out to them and explained that I was too weak to get up on my own. I asked if they could get me a chair to use to help me stand up. I honestly don't remember if they opened a classroom door and pulled a chair out for me to use (for some reason pulling myself up with the leverage was doable, compared to pushing off the ground which was not), or if they directly helped me up themselves. Either way, I was relieved that they came by and helped.

I tried not to go anywhere alone after that for some time.

Even though I missed a lot of school during that first year, my curiosity never stopped. Treatment became a unique classroom, teaching me lessons I never expected. I was always fascinated by science and focused on everything I could learn through my treatment. Here are just some of the things that I have learned about science from having cancer:

Chemotherapy attacks fast-growing cells, which is why hair is lost (among other issues).

The frequency and volume of infused medicine is dangerous for a leukemia patient's veins, so a central line is surgically inserted (mine was a port).

Low Calcium or Potassium can cause stroke-like spasms in the joints.

Leukemia cells don't fight infection, they just reproduce. They also live longer than healthy white blood cells.

Learning these scientific details gave me a deeper understanding of what was happening in my body and why treatment was so intense. But beyond the facts, it was the emotional and mental journey that shaped me most.

If you're just starting treatment or have been recently diagnosed, hearing about all the treatments, side effects, and struggles might feel overwhelming or even scary. I never thought I would be able to go a day without thinking about cancer. It consumed my every waking minute. But then, one day, I realized I hadn't thought about it in a while. You grow so much through the experience. When you're in treatment, trying to look ahead can seem like an eternity. That's because you realize how uncertain the future is. No one is promised tomorrow. I would be so jealous (which is not something I usually am) of people at the end of their treatment. It seemed so far for me, and I would think, "I'll never get there." But then you do … and time flies. Time goes by too quickly.

One way or another, you'll get through. You have so much living, experience, and trauma squeezed into a short amount of time. Can I promise everything will be okay? Unfortunately, no. But I do believe attitude and how you approach this can make a difference. There are certainly things I shouldn't have survived. But I am stubborn. My journey taught me that stubbornness isn't a flaw; it's a lifeline. So if you're reading this and facing your own fight, know this: you are stronger than you think. Keep pushing forward—you can do this.

Chapter 3
Side Effects

Disclaimer: This is not an exhaustive list of every side effect I encountered (not even taking into account the ones mentioned in the previous chapter). That would have been boring and waaaaay too much information. But this gives a good picture of what I endured.

Having cancer was the *"easy"* part.

I know how that sounds, but in many ways, it was true. If there was even a slight chance of a medication causing a rare complication, I was usually the one it happened to.

I got into the habit of reading the list of "possible side effects" for every drug I was given, trying to prepare myself for what might come. But anticipation didn't offer much protection. Eventually, the doctors stopped telling me all the potential reactions. They were concerned I might be *willing* myself into symptoms just by expecting them. I don't know if that theory held any weight, but I developed most of them anyway.

Some side effects I remember vividly. Others are hazy—lost to the fog of treatment or pain. Some come back only when something triggers a memory or someone reminds me.

The more immediate and physical reactions, or ones that needed procedural interventions, were the hardest to forget. Like during a short stretch of time when my blood sugar was all over the place due to chemo—skyrocketing one moment, crashing the next.

The low blood sugar episodes were scary. The highs didn't affect me as noticeably—at least not compared to everything else going on. Once, I felt unusually tired while visitors were in the room. I kept "falling asleep" mid-sentence, then jerking awake and trying to talk again. Over and over. We later realized I wasn't falling asleep at all—I was *passing out* from low levels. That discovery made me feel slightly better. I'd been embarrassed that someone had come all that way to visit, and I couldn't even stay conscious to talk to them. Turns out it wasn't just me being rude—I was literally losing consciousness.

At one point I had a tube inserted through my nose to help manage the levels (a "nasogastric tube" that was used to temporarily be able to get liquids and medications directly into my stomach at a controlled rate and faster than I could drink on my own). There very well could have been other reasons I required it—especially at my sickest points I just did what had to be done and didn't question too much—but I vividly remember the nurses using it to quickly get orange juice into me during one of my crashes.

Managing blood sugar meant testing constantly and using insulin—no easy task when your platelet counts are low (since those are what make your blood clot when your skin is punctured). Pricking my fingers often led to dramatic, disgusting gushes of blood. Once, I pricked my finger and sent a stream of blood clear across the room. A real blood-borne pathogen nightmare. Just another delightful layer to navigate. Obviously, finger pricks and insulin aren't uncommon, but when you're already juggling chemo, low blood counts, and everything else, it just added to the pile. The doctors didn't know whether the sugar issues would be temporary or permanent, so I mentally prepared for the long haul.

It was ironic: Before I was diagnosed, I'd wondered if I might have diabetes. Instead, I had cancer—and the treatment gave me the diabetes-like symptoms I was originally afraid of. Funny how life works.

And just when I thought the blood sugar rollercoaster was bad enough, I ended up in the ICU—for reasons that still aren't totally clear to me. What I *do* remember is that I was scheduled for a lumbar puncture and bone marrow aspirate. But they couldn't do either until I was stable, so the hospital put me on a strict diet: no food, no water, not even ice chips. It felt like I was asking for contraband just to get a sip of water.

I was in excruciating pain, and the thirst made it worse. As soon as I left the ICU, they did both procedures right there in my hospital room.

That ICU stay was the only time I remember being accessed directly in the wrist for an arterial line. It was agony. They couldn't get it right at first. With my low platelets, blood was everywhere—the bed, the floor. And the resulting bruises stretched from my wrist to elbow and lasted for weeks.

That gave me a new level of respect—not just for the extraordinary people who care for patients in those moments, but for the patients themselves. You can't fully understand what someone is going through until you watch it closely … or live it.

That deeper compassion stuck with me. But unfortunately, it didn't mean things were about to get any easier.

Not very far into treatment, I was hit with what had to be a side effect of the medication—though, at the time, no one could say exactly what it was.

It started with a single welt on my left leg, just below the knee. It was pink—almost red—and felt hot to the touch. Painful, too. *Very* painful. I thought maybe I'd bumped into something and forgotten about it. I bruised easily, and even more so with low blood counts, so that wouldn't have been unusual. But this was on the inside of my knee—an odd place to injure without noticing. Then I touched it. The heat radiating from it was unsettling. This wasn't a normal bruise.

I was at home when it first appeared. I don't remember exactly how quickly we acted—whether I spiked a fever and we rushed to the ER that night, or if I had a regular appointment the next day—but I ended up in the hospital shortly after, and by then, the sore was getting worse. Bigger. Hotter. More painful. And spreading—across both legs. Yippee, right?

The sores had a texture I didn't recognize. At first, they felt soft-silky. Much later, as they began to heal, they hardened and dried out, but in the early days, even the lightest touch sent shockwaves of pain radiating through my entire body. Naturally, that meant every doctor who came in had to press on them, examine them, and marvel at their heat. Not just warm—*hot.* I wasn't imagining it. Everyone who touched them commented on the temperature.

I was grateful that the sores stayed mostly on the tops of my legs. At least I could lie down without directly pressing on them. If they'd wrapped around my legs completely, I honestly don't know how I would've found relief.

Then came the swelling.

My legs began to fill with fluid—so much so that they looked inflated. Like balloons ready to burst. I couldn't see my ankles anymore. I couldn't bend them. I couldn't walk. My joints were surrounded by fluid, my skin stretched to the limit, with no range of motion left. In just a day or two, I stopped caring who saw me in my underwear. Pants and even blankets were out of the question. Between the swelling and the sores, even the thought of fabric brushing against my skin made me wince.

And still—*everyone* had to touch the sores. Telling them it hurt wasn't enough. They needed to see for themselves. Reactions had to be witnessed. No one had any answers. Not even the infectious disease specialist could give us an educated guess. That was *so* reassuring.

While my legs remained swollen, the nurses measured the circumference daily and kept a close watch on my weight. When the swelling finally began to subside, I lost a measurable amount of fluid weight. The welts began to shrink. Most of them faded to tiny bruise-like spots. But not the first one—the one I nicknamed the "mother sore."

The mother sore stuck around. It stayed swollen and angry looking. At its worst, it was about seven inches in diameter and rock hard. As it healed, the skin changed texture. It turned thick and tough, almost like a leathery patch—but still skin. Still alive. Not like a scab you could peel away. It was rigid, unbending. And that became a problem.

One day, long after it had "healed," I was at a movie theater when my legs gave out from under me. I fell, and the mother sore split open.

It felt like splitting a lip—except it was my knee. My knee tried to bend like a knee should, but the skin covering it couldn't flex. The whole area was too tough, too inflexible, and when it cracked, I expected blood. But instead, it leaked a clear-ish liquid. Not comforting.

Eventually, it had to be drained and biopsied. Still, no one could tell me what it was. No conclusive answers. The sore shrank slowly, and the skin softened a little over time. It eventually took on the appearance of a deep bruise.

Even now, years later, I still have a scar where that mother sore once was. It's dark, like a permanent bruise, and much larger than you'd expect from something that's technically "healed."

I've sometimes wondered if the welts were a form of chemo burn. That's what I call the scar now—a chemo burn—because, well, I don't have a better explanation. It came from chemo. It burned. It left a scar. That's good enough for me. But I'm not a doctor.

Just as the welts began to fade and the swelling finally went down, I expected—maybe even allowed myself to hope for—a return to something resembling normal. But instead, something else crept in. Something no antibiotic could fix. No amount of rest or ice packs would make it go away.

That was when we noticed I wasn't walking the way I used to.

That is when foot drop and my weak legs started. I already got into that in the last chapter (because it's almost impossible to actually separate treatment from the side effects it caused) so I won't dwell on it again.

I was starting to learn a hard truth: illness doesn't press pause on life. High school kept going. My friends kept growing up. Big moments happened with or without me. And I was doing my best to hang on—to my sense of self, to my body, to my connection with the world outside my hospital room.

One of those big moments was junior prom.

I had a date—my best friend at the time (well, my best friend who wasn't Thumper or my brother). I'd found the most beautiful dress I'd ever worn to a school dance and was genuinely excited. But, true to form, nothing came easy.

When prom day came, I wasn't getting ready at home. I was in the hospital.

And I wasn't just *in* the hospital—I was a mess. My counts were dangerously low. My body was in pain. My mouth was swollen nearly shut from mucositis. I was slipping into a kind of emotional fog that hovered somewhere between physical misery and depression. I wasn't well in any sense of the word.

Still, I was determined to go. The hospital had a system that allowed patients to leave for a few hours on a medical pass—basically checking out like a library book. I was going to take one of those passes and go to prom.

Some of my nurses were understandably alarmed. One pulled me aside and told me, very seriously, that she didn't think I would survive the dance. My immune system was so compromised that if I caught even a basic cold—let alone the flu—it would be catastrophic. She needed to make sure I understood: I was taking a real risk. Was I absolutely sure I wanted to go?

I didn't hesitate. I *had* to go.

I know how that sounds. I was never one of those "prom is everything" teenagers. But this wasn't about the dance. It was about needing something *normal*. I needed a reason to get out of bed. I needed a reminder that I still existed in the world outside of medicine and machines.

My mom had the flu and couldn't be near me. It crushed her to miss that moment—seeing me in my dress, seeing me try to reclaim some piece of teenage life—but she understood the risk. So the nurses stepped in. They helped my dad and brother get me ready. They helped me into my gown and helped me adjust my wig (which I rarely wore). They gave us a sweet little send-off, the kind that you don't forget.

They also made sure I was on every type of pain medication legally available to keep me going through the evening. I had IV meds before I was unhooked from the line, a pain patch that would absorb through my skin over time, and a handful of pills. I even had medicated "lollipops" designed to absorb through the mucus membranes. My family got quite the crash course in palliative pain relief. If anyone didn't know our medical situation, they probably would've assumed we were running some kind of underground pharmacy.

My dad and brother brought me to the pre-prom photos and picked me up when I was ready to leave. At the photo spot, I remember thinking I was smiling—pushing through the pain to look like I was enjoying myself. Later, when I saw the pictures, I realized how bad I looked. My jaw was visibly swollen, my face puffed up from the mouth sores, and I wasn't smiling at all. But I was happy—at least, as happy as someone in that much pain could be.

I couldn't open my mouth more than a sliver. Talking was torture. Eating was out of the question, which was heartbreaking because the buffet looked and smelled incredible. Even my "miracle mouthwash" wasn't enough this time. It worked best right before a meal, giving me a small window to eat—but not that night.

I was able to drink, slowly, through a straw. My date was so kind—he helped me find one and got me what I needed, since shouting over the music or walking across the room weren't options. The friends I hadn't seen in months were excited to see me and I them, and it broke my heart that I couldn't really talk to them. The sores extended so far down my throat that even speaking felt like being stabbed from the inside out.

Still, the friends who had been with me through everything—through diagnosis, treatment, hospital stays—made it as easy and special as they could. Just being at a high school prom, under the lighting and decor, surrounded by normal teenage chaos … it was magnificent.

When my excursion pass ended and I returned to the hospital, it was almost a relief. I was exhausted—physically drained and emotionally raw—but I had something I hadn't had in a while: a good memory.

That night reminded me I was still part of the world. And I came back to my hospital bed with a slightly fuller heart and a little more hope.

That prom night reminded me just how unpredictable everything had become. One moment, I was in a gown trying to smile through the pain. The next, I was back in a hospital bed in my pajamas, hooked to monitors and IVs. That back-and-forth, that constant shift between the surreal and the ordinary, had become my new normal. Especially when it came to timing—because if something was going to go wrong, it was guaranteed to happen after hours.

Nothing ever happened during business hours, when doctors were easy to reach and the clinic was open. No, the real fun always began late at night, over weekends, or on holidays. And more often than not, it started with a fever. Any fever meant something was likely brewing inside me—some infection or complication—so we won ourselves a trip to the emergency room. Again.

Now, let me be clear: I have nothing against emergency room staff. They do incredible work under pressure, with wildly unpredictable situations. But when you're on a highly specific treatment plan—like chemotherapy—there's a real comfort in working with people who understand the protocol. That's where the oncology floor shined.

On the oncology floor, I was treated like a VIP. The nurses and doctors knew me, and I knew them. Everything was streamlined. I could just rattle off my date of birth and name—like a song I'd memorized—and they'd give me meds, take blood, or adjust my treatment. Easy. Efficient. Familiar.

In the ER? Whole different universe.

There, I was just another unknown patient. It didn't matter how sick I looked or that I was clearly mid-treatment. I had to verify every detail of my medical history—over and over and over. Each new person who walked in (and there were always many) asked me the same questions, often while I was half-conscious, nauseated, or writhing in pain. I get the need for caution and protocol, especially at intake, but at a certain point I just wanted to yell, "Read my chart!"

I wasn't checking into the hospital as a spa retreat. I was there because I felt horrible. Being interrogated like I was trying to sneak in for free snacks didn't exactly help.

I remember one particular ER visit where they couldn't even locate my doctor in the system. For a brief moment, I had an existential crisis. Was I imagining this entire thing? Had I created a phantom doctor and made up months of chemo? But no—they eventually found him. Turned out I had a fever and what I *thought* was an ear infection. The funny part? Every single person I saw asked me what was wrong with my eye.

"Nothing," I insisted. "It's my *ear*."

They kept staring at my face, confused. "Are you sure? Looks like something's up with your eye."

Well—guess what? The next day, I woke up with pinkeye.

Experiences like that reminded me just how important it was to stay actively involved in my own care. That's why, from very early on in treatment, I kept notebooks close by. I always had one within reach.

I'd jot down questions to ask doctors during rounds or at the clinic. I tracked my blood sugar levels, my temperatures, and any strange symptoms that cropped up. It gave me a tiny sense of control in a world where very little felt controllable. And it helped make sure I didn't forget important details when I finally had someone to talk to.

Looking back through those notebooks now is like flipping through a chronicle of survival. One thing that stands out—besides the content—is how my handwriting changed over time. It started off neat, the way I'd always written. But as the weeks and months went on, the writing got sloppier, shakier, almost illegible. Holding a pen had become difficult. It wasn't just the pain—it was the coordination, the grip. My hands didn't work like they used to.

Even now, I have to really concentrate if I want to write neatly. I *can* do it—but my hand cramps much faster than before. And I'm not talking about the old "I've been writing for an hour" kind of cramp. I mean sharp, sudden, throbbing spasms. The kind that come after just a few lines. The kind that makes you drop your pen like it's electrified.

Hand charley horses, I call them.

Remember back in school—this one's for my middle-aged audience (kidding … kind of)—writing pages of notes would eventually give you that dull, achy fatigue in your hand? Now, I get a full-blown hand spasm just from holding a fork too tightly or gripping a shopping bag. The muscles seize, and the only solution is to let go—drop whatever I'm holding and wait for it to pass. It's annoying. It's unpredictable. And it's just one of the lasting gifts chemo left behind.

On the topic of charley horses … have you ever had one? That sudden, jarring, completely uncontrollable contraction of a muscle—usually at the most inconvenient time possible? If you have, then you understand why the term "charley horse" feels like a gross understatement. I also had them in my legs. And these weren't minor cramps. These were total, muscle-seizing, leg-paralyzing attacks that left me breathless.

The spasms were mostly in my right calf, and they came with zero warning. No twinge. No tightening. Just *BAM*—pain. My entire calf muscle would lock, twist, and contract like it was trying to rip itself off the bone. The first few seconds felt like an electric shock. Then came the burning. Then the wait. Because that's all I *could* do—wait it out. Thirty seconds of agony feels like thirty minutes. You lose track of time when your leg is trying to self-destruct.

There wasn't a position that prevented them—lying down didn't help. I'd get them in my sleep. I'd get them in the bathtub. I'd get them in water aerobics.

Yes. Water aerobics. I took that class … in college.

I took it because I needed a kinesthetic class, and running or jumping was off the table. My only other classmate was a sweet, elderly nun who lived on campus, and honestly, it was one of the most wholesome college experiences I had. But it wasn't my first choice. I'd originally wanted to take an acting course to fulfill the requirement, but it was only offered Monday afternoons—and guess who had treatment then? My college schedule had to revolve around my chemo calendar. While most of my classmates were planning electives around sleep schedules or extracurriculars, I was planning mine around treatment windows.

Balancing treatment with daily life wasn't just exhausting—it was emotionally disorienting. For every side effect I expected, five more came out of nowhere. And every new pain brought fresh anxiety. Each unusual twinge, every unfamiliar ache, made me wonder: *Is this something new, or something old returning? Is this the beginning of something worse?*

That's a weight that still lingers.

Even now, long after treatment, I don't feel entirely safe in my own body. I live with the constant awareness that something could go wrong again—that something is *waiting* to go wrong. It's like having a shadow that never quite disappears. A quiet voice that whispers, *You've been too lucky. You're on borrowed time. It's just a matter of when.*

Late effects. Secondary cancers. Scares that might not show up for years. I try not to dwell on it, but that doesn't mean it's nonexistent. I've had unexplained chest pains. Tests came back inconclusive, which sounds like good news, except I know my heart is one of the areas they monitor for long-term damage. Because with the drugs I was given, cardiac problems later in life are—if not expected—then not exactly a surprise.

I worry that something could get missed. That symptoms will be dismissed because I'm "too young" or because the late effects aren't fully understood. The truth is, modern long-term survivorship for childhood leukemia hasn't been around long enough for us to know everything. We're still the first waves on the shore. We're the case studies in progress.

And I've already seen what happens when things are overlooked. It took forever for doctors to correctly diagnose the AVN (avascular necrosis) in my shoulders. It wasn't anyone's fault—it was just too easy to miss the dots that connected it to my treatment history. That's what keeps me awake some nights. The "what ifs." What if I ignore a symptom I shouldn't? What if something small is actually the first clue to something big?

These fears don't control me anymore. Not like they used to. But they're still there, quiet and stubborn. I still flinch when pain hits in a new place. I still wake up wondering if today is the day my calf decides to revolt again. I still brace myself for the next blood draw, the next check-up, the next wave of unknowns.

But I've also learned this: **life doesn't come with guarantees.**

So I take the good days as they come. I laugh when it doesn't hurt too much—even if it feels wildly inappropriate. I cry when I need to. I wear my scars like the badges of honor they are. Some are visible. Some aren't. But they're all part of me.

And I'm still here.

And that counts for something.

Heck … It counts for everything.

PART TWO

What Kept Me Going

Chapter 4
My Hero

Everyone deserves a hero. Someone to look up to, that makes them smile, and gives them something to keep fighting for.

A huge aspect of my life that bridged the gap from pre- to post-diagnosis was my love, respect, and admiration for Johnny Depp—someone who brought me joy during some of the darkest moments. It's hard to explain exactly why I love someone so deeply, and despite years of trying, I'm not sure *I'll* ever fully understand my infatuation with him. I just know it's a form of true love. He brings immeasurable joy to my life, and I want nothing but the best for him (even while knowing that has absolutely nothing to do with me).

I have a rather unique experience with Johnny Depp and my "celebrity crush" on him. The first thing people tend to know about me is that he's my favorite actor (it's difficult to "know" me and not see that), but few can appreciate why, or to what DEPPth ... sorry ... *depth* ... I admire him. His presence in my life shaped more than just my entertainment choices—it became a key part of who I was during a time of upheaval. Even if others didn't always get it, Johnny Depp was a hero to me, and that connection was unshakeable. After *Pirates of the Caribbean* came out, I eagerly tracked down each of his major films, becoming completely hooked. His ability to transform into unforgettable characters mesmerized me, and, beyond his on-screen talent, I respected the man himself.

As my admiration grew, Johnny became more than just a distant celebrity—he seeped into the fabric of my everyday life. I thought about him constantly (not in a creepy way), and it showed—anyone who sees my car immediately knows I'm a fan. Without giving too much personal information away (as if I haven't already), there's something that screams "this is Katie's car!" when you see it. If you ever come across my car, you'll know *exactly* what I mean. It's adorable when someone comes up and tells me about "this car they saw in the parking lot, and have I seen it?" (Referring to my car.) It takes restraining every sarcastic bone in my body to answer with a straight face that the car is mine. Like, who else in the vicinity would be more of a Johnny Depp fan than I am to have that car? (Unless I'm somewhere such as a Hollywood Vampires concert, which even then, a friend I was meeting in person for the first time *still* immediately knew it was me by my car.)

When illness entered my life, Johnny's movies transformed from mere entertainment to a vital refuge. Watching his films became my escape, transporting me to different worlds and helping me forget pain and fear, if only for a little while. It was magical. No pain medicine ever did for me what Johnny did. And following the production of his current films gave me hope for what was to come. Those were the moments I would plan on a future (something I didn't do much of once I was diagnosed). I had every intention of seeing his movies that hadn't been released yet. No way was I going to miss a single one.

The release of *Sweeney Todd* kept me happily distracted (with interviews to watch and magazine articles to read). When the movie came out in December of 2007, it was the first one I went to see in the cinema since being diagnosed. I had recently been let out of the hospital, and my friends went with me like we did whenever a Johnny movie premiered.

Sweeney Todd was instantly my favorite movie. For many reasons. It was directed by my favorite director (Tim Burton), Johnny sang (for the first time that the world got to hear), it had some of my other favorite actors in it such as Alan Rickman and Helena Bonham Carter. And it was just *really* good.

It came to DVD on my 17th birthday (remember physical media?), and I was in the hospital getting chemo. That evening, my friends came up and threw me a little party. My family gave me the DVD and we watched it together. My parents gave me a book on the production of *Sweeney Todd* I thoroughly enjoyed. The behind-the-scenes images and information allowed me to pretend I was there on set. That has been my craziest dream since I discovered Johnny. I'd love to work on a film with him in any capacity. I later decided that I would ask Johnny to sign this book when I met him during my Make-A-Wish.

Before *Sweeney Todd* came out, I was enjoying the small pot pies the cafeteria would have. That was all I ate for the longest time. Once the film came out (if you are unfamiliar with the plot, it involves people being killed and baked into mini meat pies), I could no longer stomach the cafeteria pies. So … that was fun. I had to find something else to eat that didn't make me think I was eating people. (*Because that is called "cannibalism"* … Nope. I'm not finishing that *Charlie and the Chocolate Factory* reference.)

Before I was diagnosed (but I had already been following the production of the movie), I heard that Johnny's daughter had become very ill while he was filming *Sweeney Todd*. She was not doing well for a while, and Johnny almost stepped down from his role. I learned a lot about children's hospitals at that point, as he never left her bedside. She was treated at a hospital in London, which is an incredible hospital I support now in Johnny's honor. Thankfully, his daughter ended up being okay.

When I was told I qualified for Make-A-Wish, my first reaction was disbelief—*"but that's for sick kids."* Maybe I didn't fully accept how sick I was, or maybe denial was just easier. But then, almost immediately, my mind raced to one thought: *"Can I finally meet Johnny Depp?"* The chance to meet my hero suddenly felt within reach. I had been a fan for four years at that point (which, 25% of your life is an eternity) and had a strong desire to act with him; at the very least, *meet* him. I also knew that he had granted other children's wishes to meet him. I was told "yes." It might take a while since he was popular and busy, but it would likely happen. I was added to the list of kids waiting to meet him. Johnny became a great part of the inspiration I needed to get through the challenges cancer threw at me.

The wish process officially began one evening when two volunteer Wish Granters from Make-A-Wish came to our house. Nice people. They explained the process and got the ball rolling by filling out paperwork. They asked me if I had thought about what my wish would be. *Only every single day, even before I knew I'd get one!*

I wanted to meet Johnny [Depp]. (Whenever I have to clarify which "Johnny" I'm talking about, I can tell that the person I'm speaking with doesn't know me yet. His last name is implied when I say "Johnny.")

"Are you sure?"

Um ... yes. 1000%.

"No matter how long you have to wait?"

Yup.

"Do you have a backup wish if this one doesn't pan out?"

There was no way I would accept that Johnny *wouldn't* pan out. This was my chance ... possibly my *only* chance ... to meet him. I could think of "other" wishes that would have been nice, but none could hold a candle to meeting my hero. I would only allow myself to consider alternatives if Johnny was absolutely off the table.

With my heart set on meeting Johnny, I knew I couldn't consider any other wish—so everything was officially in motion. I don't recall seeing those volunteers again through my wish process. Hopefully they're well. My wish was a waiting game for the next four years, until everything happened all at once. And I mean *all at once*.

While the waiting stretched on for years, the thought of my wish kept me going. Even though I had no idea when the call would come saying it was my turn to meet Johnny, this kept me looking forward to something. At any minute, my family could be told my dream was about to come true, and I'd be whisked off to who knew where around the world to meet him. It could be down the street from me, the other side of the country, or the opposite side of the world. Wherever he was when he had the time to grant the wishes of the next kids waiting for him.

Every big event, particularly around the time of film premieres (which I was following anyway), I was on high alert. With as busy of a schedule as an A-list celebrity has, I thought the best time to fit wish granting in would be when he already had commitments to make public appearances, even big TV show appearances. Each time those would approach, I would be lying if I said I didn't hope our phone would ring, forever changing our life. I had crazy daydreams that I would meet him on a fun talk show. Because, how cool would it be to not only meet him, but see a show filmed live? I also dreamed that maybe we'd go to the next *Pirates of the Caribbean* set (maybe even be an extra …), or premiere. But in the end, it didn't matter if I met Johnny at the end of my driveway for five minutes. Johnny was the wish. And I was 100% okay with that.

But when the first call came, it was not at all what I was expecting. I didn't even know it had come … until later. That wasn't the best part of my cancer journey. It was not the easiest in terms of side effects, and I was quite ill.

That call wasn't what I had imagined at all. My family was out to eat one day when I was out of the hospital … getting pancakes … and they told me that Make-A-Wish had contacted them. We were given the chance to meet Johnny. At first, I didn't know where the conversation was going, and I half expected to be told my wish was about to happen.

My parents had been given a few hours to decide, but they ultimately said no, because I was too sick and wouldn't have been able to enjoy, or possibly even make it *to*, the meet. That hurt. I was getting older and might not have had another chance to meet him through my wish. (You had to qualify for your wish before you were eighteen, but had until your twenty-first birthday in order for your wish to be granted.)

That was as hopeless as I'd felt in terms of my wish. I had wanted to meet Johnny for so long, and so badly, but my one shot to finally do that might have just passed. I knew my parents had my best interest at heart, and they really wanted me to enjoy my wish. But in my heart, I was afraid I had just lost my only chance. As difficult as it was, I tried to keep the faith that what is meant to be, will be. (Don't you hate when everything is going wrong, and people tell you that? That everything will work out in the end? It should provide comfort, but sometimes it feels like it lets the wind out of what's left in your sails.)

I tried to keep my chin up, and wished harder … even if it didn't make sense.

We received a letter while Johnny was filming *Pirates of the Caribbean 4* in Hawaii, just to check in and let us know I was still on the list. When the message first came, I thought it was going to be a "come to the set of your favorite franchise to hang out in a state your parents always said was beautiful" memo. Alas, it was not. But things will work out in the end, right?

I will always remember, a few months later I was working at the local ice cream parlor, and *Pirates of the Caribbean 4* was having its premiere in Disneyland, California. *Come on!* That HAD to be a perfect spot to bring Make-A-Wish kids! Down to the minute the premiere was scheduled to start, I kept checking my phone in case my parents called saying we had to get to the airport … Remember, I'm not the brightest bulb in the box. Clearly getting to the airport (forget packing!), flying, and getting to Disneyland would take WAY longer than the actual premiere and we would have missed it anyway. But … *hope.* Hope was all I had at times, and I wasn't going to let any of it go.

My college offered special services for students in situations such as mine. I chose the school I went to for several reasons. It was well known for being good for education and science (and becoming a Chemistry teacher was my plan). It was close to CCMC. And it was a small school. A school where I would be more than just a number, and someone would realize if I didn't show up to class. We wanted someone to be aware of my history and treatment plan, who we would be able to contact and help me work with my professors if I ever had to miss time from class for medical reasons.

My first year, I had told the person in charge of the special services that my Make-A-Wish might be granted at any time, and we might not have much notice (as that's how celebrity wishes tend to work). She said we would figure it out when the time came. At the beginning of my second and third years, I touched base with her again, just to remind her that I was still waiting for Johnny. Shortly after the third time, I sent her a "this is not a drill" email. I was off to meet Johnny and would miss a week of classes. She was great and got a memo out to all my professors. All but one was tremendously accommodating for this once-in-a-lifetime opportunity I had no direct control over.

I will always remember the day my family came to tell me it was finally going to happen. It was a Thursday—the same day I'd just attempted (unsuccessfully) to start an improv night at school. My family had called earlier and asked if they could stop by afterward and visit. I thought that was a little odd because I would be going home the following day (like I did every Friday), but why not? They said they would come by when my dad got out of work (or something like that). My brother, D.J., was driving the family van (because that was *the* family vehicle back then). My mom was in the passenger seat, and my dad was in the back. They parked in my dorm's lot, and I went up to the passenger side window to say hi to my mom (and Thumper). I whacked my head on the rain guard, and my family laughed. Good old fun. Laughing at each other's pain and conceivable concussion … I got in the back seat next to my dad. Thumper gave me a little wrapped box, which I immediately recognized as a bead box from a small store we had occasionally frequented. My mom and I had started charm bracelets for special moments and owned a few beads to commemorate some significant milestones. We also were quite friendly with the owner of the store. I was, at first, a little sad they went without me, as I really enjoyed seeing the owner.

Then I opened the box.

I was confused and didn't quite understand. It was a very special bead I had picked to get *after* I had met Johnny. The bead said "dreams really do come true."

My mom asked if I knew what it was. *Yes. It was the bead I wanted to get* after *I met Johnny. I don't think that has happened yet. Unless this chemo brain was getting worse …*

My mom said, "Are you ready?"

You better not be joking.

"Yes!!! When?"

We would be leaving in 48 hours for London and meeting him on the set of *Dark Shadows* (which I thought had wrapped already). For the first time I could remember, I cried happy tears. I was overwhelmed with the greatest feeling of joy I had ever experienced. Mixed with that was an immense sense of relief. I had hit rock bottom of my "meeting Johnny" hope. With only a few months remaining until my twenty-first birthday, I had accepted that Make-A-Wish would not be the way I was going to meet him. I was running out of time. Being given a wish was like a magic wand that was going to make my improbable goal of meeting him come true. But with each passing day, that was looking less and less likely. But now … it was happening! And in just a few days! I cried for probably twenty minutes.

And it just kept getting better.

D.J. said Johnny would only meet me if Tim Burton could be with him. *WHAT?* Tim is my favorite director, and I never even dared to dream that I would meet him, too.

Once I stopped crying for a moment, I realized that London was in another country. (I will always be the first to say I'm not that quick.) I had never been there and didn't think anyone else in my family had been, either. I'd only ever spent a few hours outside of America, on a day trip from California to Mexico. As far as I knew, I was the only one in my family with a valid passport. I had gotten one the previous year when my college had done an event to promote studying abroad, and I thought it would help as a form of identification to apply for jobs or travel domestically. At that point, I did not have plans to ever leave the country. Who would have guessed that I would have needed it to go on my Make-A-Wish? I immediately thought that my family would not be able to come with me on the trip if they didn't also have passports. If they had to pass this time around … *again* … there most certainly would not be another shot before I aged out of being able to receive a wish. This was *it*.

"Wait, do you have passports? Because I am going!" This was nonnegotiable, even if I had to call Make-A-Wish back and beg them to let me go on my own. I was so considerate to think of ditching my family that quickly …

I'm not going to lie … that would probably still be my reaction today if this happened all over again. I could always send a postcard home to them … *Priorities.* Meeting my hero was what mattered. It would be awesome if my family could come, but … *Priorities.*

My family had been in secret contact with Make-A-Wish for some time, and they had been given the idea that my wish was likely to be granted abroad at the last minute (so getting passports was a *very* good idea). My family's passports had apparently arrived in the nick of time. Because my wish was going to be granted in another country (England), the UK chapter and my local chapter had to communicate back and forth to get everything arranged. With the time difference, that was a logistical nightmare.

My Make-A-Wish chapter (most of the people on the staff) helped to get all the details ironed out and arranged. From the flights, to the hotel, to the limo transportation, to the enhancements, to the wheelchair for my mom (she started needing one to get around long distances during my treatment) at every step of the way, to coordinating the meet-and-greet. My family had been given the official word that the wish was going to happen the day before I was told. Later on, when I came back to Make-A-Wish to volunteer, everyone who helped on my wish remembered me as the "Johnny Depp wish." All wish kids are treated like royalty, as they should be.

I wasn't allowed to post about meeting Johnny online before it happened. There wasn't as much online activity in 2011 compared to nowadays, but that was still difficult when

I wanted to scream from the rooftops: "I'M MEETING JOHNNY DEPP!"

So, what did I do instead? I couldn't actually get onto the roof, but I ran around my dorm, *actually* screaming at the top of my lungs to all my friends (and some random people, too). My poor roommate. I stormed into our room, screamed I was going to meet Johnny (likely incoherently and startling her), then cried. Then I screamed again and kept crying hot and happy tears. It was a roller coaster of emotions.

When I eventually calmed down enough to be slightly coherent, I kept running around the floor to anyone I could find. I told my resident assistant (RA) that I was going to be gone the following week, and she gave me some tips on what to wear and bring to Europe (apparently it rains a lot … so I would need an umbrella). *Oh, yeah.* I would have to pack for another country! I next went to one of my best friends. She also told me to bring an umbrella. Nothing was going to rain on my parade. Not even *actual* rain. I love how supportive my friends were of how ecstatic I was. Even if they couldn't comprehend exactly what meeting Johnny meant to me, they knew it was inexplicably important to me and shared in my happiness.

When I got back to my room, I tried on just about every article of clothing I had, because I had to select the perfect outfit to meet Johnny in. This was going to be the best day of my life, and I had to look as good as possible. (I'm normally in jeans and a T-shirt when I'm not at work, but I wanted to wear something a little nicer for what I hoped would include a photo with Johnny I would be looking at for the rest of my life.) I eventually picked out the outfit (knowing full well I would only wear it one more time, on the day of my wish … I've been assured that not wearing clothes you've worn on super special occasions is a semi-normal thing to do).

After I had run around, screamed, cried … I was a little exhausted but still full of emotion (and a tad bit of disbelief). I posted a few hearts on Facebook, because I couldn't say anything. This was also when I emailed the person in charge of special services at the school.

I have zero recollection of school the next day. But when I got home, we packed. It was a full-circle moment. The last time we were scrambling to pack together was the day I was diagnosed before going to the hospital. This time, we were off on the trip of a lifetime.

My family had not been on a "let's get on a plane and stay in a hotel" vacation in years, let alone across the pond to a foreign country, so it should have been a touch overwhelming for someone like me. I over-plan and over-pack … normally. My family was stressed (and justifiably, as usually I would also have been right there with them). But for some reason, I was at ease. We had been informed that Make-A-Wish had taken care of everything. They had booked the flights and hotel, a limo was going to pick us up right at our house to bring us to the airport, we were going to be picked up at the airport and brought to our hotel, someone would collect us the day of the wish to bring us to and from the meet, and we would be returned to the airport and back home when we landed. We were also given what

Make-A-Wish calculated as expenses for the days we would be on the trip (which seemed like way more than my frugal family would need), so theoretically we would not have to pay for food or souvenirs from our pockets. This was an extreme relief for me, because I didn't want an unexpected trip to put any further financial strain on our family, and we *didn't* need to pay for anything ourselves! And … I was going to get to meet Johnny Depp. This was a win-win-win situation that seemed perfect. There was nothing for me to worry about.

We also had a temporary, and unofficial, itinerary. "Katie's wish to meet Johnny Depp." Seeing those words on my wish packet made it real. The information on the flights and hotel was there. The more important details (on the greet itself) were not finalized. But it was going to happen on Monday, the 19th of September. The day I had been waiting so long for. We would get the final itinerary once we got to London. Or, that was the plan.

A shiny black stretch limousine came and collected us at our house that Saturday. The smell of the leather seats greeted us as we slid into the back. Our luggage was packed into the trunk, and we were off.

We were driven to an airport in New York. It was exciting from the start. We drove past landmarks that were from one of the World's Fairs (apparently my mom had attended), and I knew from the climax of *Men in Black.*

When we arrived at the airport, we checked in and made our way to the terminal. Since we had essentially no time to research or get foreign currency, we figured that out while we were waiting for our flight. There was a service that was basically a prepaid debit card, which would allow you to make purchases in any currency. We got a few cards so our funds were not in one location, and I felt super powerful when I was given authority to hold on to one. Once we were in London, we would take turns on who would use their card, so it was as if we were rotating who was "treating" to dinner (it's the small things in my family).

As we were sitting and waiting for our flight, the boarding time kept getting pushed back. I remember that our flight was originally in the evening (maybe about 7 pm), but not extremely late. Boarding kept getting bumped without a word from anyone working at the airport, or a reason on why. At first, I was okay. It didn't matter when we got on the plane … **I was going to get to meet Johnny.** Literally nothing could bother me.

After about two hours of pushing the time back, I started to get nervous. *What if our ride from the airport in London didn't know about the delay and left without us?*

Eventually, we got on the plane. We were now taking off in the wee hours of Sunday morning. My family was scattered around the plane, because the tickets had been booked at the last minute. (There is some disagreement on how we were seated, because it has been several years and this was not the *most* important part of the trip … Heck, I would have swum across the Atlantic Ocean, aka "The Pond," if they'd asked me to! And I don't know how to swim.) I think I sat next to someone in my family, and the other two were separated. Whether or not those two ended up together (by trading seats or not) will forever remain a mystery, as everyone in my family has a different recollection of this.

My dad asked a flight attendant why the flight had been delayed, and they responded that it had been struck by lightning on the previous trip, so it had to be carefully assessed. They could have said the plane had crashed into a million pieces on the ride over and had to be reassembled like a LEGO set missing its direction booklet, and I would *still* be trusting it to get me to London at that point. (My parents felt a tad differently.) The clock was ticking, and I had to get there to see Johnny!

Once we finally got off the ground, I watched different films on the seatback screen. Sleep was not an option. The one I remember is *Pirates of the Caribbean 4*. The whole time, I smiled from ear to ear. I was *actually* going to meet *the* Captain Jack Sparrow in approximately 24 hours. AND … It was going to be International Talk like a Pirate Day! How perfect was that? This was one of those moments where everything was aligning better than I could have imagined. Every single time I had felt heartbroken over the fact I thought I wasn't going to meet him … every missed chance … it was all leading up to this. It was happening, and it seemed beyond perfect.

My family regrouped when the plane touched down in London. My mom had been telling (just about everyone she came across, because she was super excited for me) someone on the plane that we were on our way to meet Johnny. That person had met Johnny before and raved about what a lovely person he was. The gentleman who pushed my mom's wheelchair at the airport also said he had met Johnny a few times around the airport. It seemed as if everyone we came into contact with had seen Johnny at least once before. *How do people just run into Johnny Depp?* I had been trying to meet him for eight years and had to use my once-in-a-lifetime wish to do so (which I would do a million times over). It was taunting me how he seemed to be everywhere except wherever I was (some of my good friends who I only met because of our shared appreciation for Johnny joke that he must have tracking devices on us). But I remained focused on what mattered: I *was* meeting him—tomorrow!

We collected our luggage and were driven to our hotel. Or, as close to our hotel as the driver could get. There was something going on in the streets of London that day, and we were right near the Tower of London.

When we went to check in, we were supposed to pick up the official itinerary with the schedule for the next day (which was the actual wish day). The package had not arrived, but we were assured that it should come, at the very latest, by the next morning before our experience.

Up the lift to our adjoining rooms we went. Did I mention it was my parents' anniversary the day we arrived in London? *Oops.* My wish sort of overshadowed it that year. In my parents' room was a bottle of champagne. It was a nice surprise since we weren't able to truly celebrate with how jet-lagged we were. My brother and I shared a room, which was next door. We called the local Make-A-Wish chapter to let them know we didn't have the final itinerary. They were very nice and told us what time the limo was going to pick us up the next morning and to check if the package had arrived before we left (as it was supposed to have come already since it had been overnighted).

We had no idea what was around the area of our hotel and didn't want to explore too much that evening since the following day was going to be epic. Plus, we were exhausted from traveling. We wandered around and found a Burger King nearby. Dinner was served. We're *so* adventurous.

I went to sleep knowing that that was the final time I'd go to bed and be able to dream about what meeting Johnny would be like before it actually happened.

The next morning was go-time. I had butterflies in my stomach. I was ready. I had my *Sweeney Todd* book I would ask Johnny to sign, a rock with a message I had contemplated giving to Johnny, a pen, and some blank paper in case any kid needed something to sign. (There would be other wish kids who were on the wait list to meet him there.) Thumper also came in my backpack. He went everywhere important with me. In my pocket was a small clear trinket with a flying pig. My mom and I each had one, and we would make wishes on them (mine was that I would finally meet Johnny). The whole idea that it would happen "when pigs fly" and there was a pig flying in this token made anything seem possible.

We went down to breakfast before the limo was due to pick us up. Breakfast was included in our hotel stay. There was a continental one, and you could also order special dishes off a menu. That day, we didn't know we could order off the menu, but found plenty at the continental one. I don't think I could have eaten much that morning anyway. The butterflies were making knots in my stomach.

After we were finished, we waited for the limo in the lobby. We checked to see if the itinerary had arrived ... nope. *Okay* ... So we waited without it.

And waited.

And waited.

And then waited some more.

If my anxiety was a volcano, it started heating up when the limo was around 15 minutes late. *Stuff happens ... It'll be here ...*

That volcano started smoking when the limo was a half hour late.

Lava started streaming down the sides of that volcano when the limo was 45 minutes late.

There was a full eruption of the volcano when the limo was an hour late.

The entire volcano exploded from the inside, sending shrapnel of igneous rock soaring for miles when the limo was an hour and fifteen minutes late.

I was such a pleasure during the ninety minutes we waited for the limousine to arrive past its scheduled time. I tried so hard to stay calm. *Traffic. They're coming.* Then, it got to the point that maybe they *weren't* coming. And what if they didn't? What if they didn't get us there in time for the greet? Would Johnny ever even know I was supposed to be there? The greet would have gone on as planned for the other kids, and then what? Make-A-Wish got us to London. There was no way they would send us somewhere again if something messed up with this greet, right? And even if they could, I was so close to aging out. There was zero chance they owed us anything for a limo driver not getting us to the wish on time. I was SO CLOSE to my dream, and I was going to miss out. I should have expected this as it was my track record until that point whenever meeting Johnny was concerned. Get almost, but not all the way, there. So close, but worlds apart.

Eventually, my family scraped me off the ceiling when the limo actually arrived, and my blood pressure started to come out of the stratosphere. There had been something that caused the driver to have difficulties getting around. That was a very valid excuse, as they were driving a stretch limo around the narrow streets of old London.

I was immediately excited again now that the wish was back in gear. I was still a tad nervous that I would miss the meet, but more confident that I would still get to at least *see* Johnny.

My family settled in, and we were off to Buckinghamshire. As we were getting close, we were driving by nice green fields and cute houses in the countryside. We then drove by a sign that made everything real. It said "Pinewood Studios." I couldn't believe we were there and going to be heading inside. Some of my favorite movies had been filmed there, and (at least at the time of writing this) the general public was not allowed to tour the facility. Maybe that will change one day.

I'm very glad D.J. had the idea and was quick enough to take a photo of me in front of the sign as the limo drove by. Considering I take horrible photos, that one didn't come out *that* bad.

We were brought as far as possible before we had to change into a smaller vehicle to enter the property. We were then taken to Stage A, where we signed agreements that we would not take our own photos or share anything about the film being made online before it was released. That film was being kept under wraps more so than most others I had followed. There weren't many pictures that had been released, and not much was known at that point. I would have my photo taken with Johnny and that would be sent to us after the movie came out the following year. At that point, they could have asked me to promise my first-born child in order to gain access to the greet and I might have agreed. I let my brother (who has a law degree) read the agreement. I signed and asked what next.

When we got past that point, we had a family photo taken. I realized later it was one of my favorite photographers, as he's the one who has taken some of my favorite behind-the-scenes images of Johnny on different projects; he's an unbelievable artist.

Next, we were brought to the group of kids and their families being given a tour of the props by the property master of the film. They were on the last item, and I was a little sad we had missed it. I had always been fascinated by props used in films and had never been so close to real ones. And props Johnny touched? Even better.

Oh, well. Johnny is the reason we're here. Anything else is a bonus.

The rest of the group was taken off to lunch and a tour of the water tanks used in filming. We were told we would get to see the tank later, and the property master was nice enough to take us through the props he had shown already. Since everyone else had already seen them, it was just my family getting a personal tour. There were so many cool things we got to see and some that I got to hold. Even though I didn't know what everything was being used for in the movie, once I saw the final project later it was awesome to know I had seen the props. The level of detail on them was outstanding. He showed us Barnabas's (Johnny's character in the movie) wolf-head cane, umbrella, sunglasses (which barely fit my head … Johnny must have a small head), and ring (which perfectly fit my pointer finger; Johnny and I are the same ring size!). I eventually realized that this was the same person who did the props on *Sweeney Todd* (my favorite film until that day, when I decided *Dark Shadows* was going to be my new favorite … even though it hadn't even wrapped yet …).

We also saw lanterns of different weights for various camera angles so some could be held longer than others, the "family car" complete with a Maine license plate (the location where *Dark Shadows* took place), models of the set, portraits, a chandelier and breakable glass, pendants of various materials for countless shots … And a treasure chest with some fake coins. I picked a few up, (pretended they were some of 882 identical pieces of cursed Aztec gold medallions as I put them back … because what *Pirates of the Caribbean* fan would I be if I hadn't?), and wanted so badly to ask to keep one (or *anything*). But at that point, I hadn't met Johnny, and did not want to get thrown out for stealing anything or offending the people being so kind with their time to show us around. So, I put every last one of the coins back, and we were brought to lunch.

Lunch was from the catering truck that the cast and crew ate from. At this point, my stomach was entirely inside out. I would be meeting Johnny at any moment. I got some pineapple upside down cake, a piece of ham, and green beans. It was packaged in a white to-go container, and we sat down in a covered area to eat. What I was able to eat was delicious. My mom (who had been seated while we got the food) had said there was someone who looked like Johnny sitting at a table near her while we were in line. I swear … if he had been right there and I missed him … That was my luck with him. It turns out, it was his stand-in.

After lunch, we returned to the soundstage to watch them film. It was too dangerous for us to be directly on set with them (they were using fire that day), so we watched through a monitor as they filmed next door. That was *fascinating*! They had to film a few seconds in each take multiple times. They would do one angle, then another. The first few were of Angelique (played by Eva Green), then it was Johnny's turn. Watching him create what I knew was going to be a part of my favorite movie, aka *cinematic history*, was magical and surreal.

At some point, we were offered snacks and drinks and told that the greet would be happening soon. I had some Cadbury chocolates, crispy M&Ms, and a fruit smoothie. My parents socialized a bit with other parents. I would have loved to talk to some of the other kids and find out what brought them to want to meet Johnny—or Tim, as some kids were there to meet Tim Burton. But I was far too nervous and in my own head at the moment. (I'm very thankful I did connect with one of the other girls afterward, and we touch base on our wishiversary each year.)

At the time, I was playing over and over what I wanted to say to Johnny and trying to make it as coherent as possible. We had been told that we would be able to ask one question (and that is all we were guaranteed). Being the kind of person I am, I tried to pack as much into that one question as I could. If we were given any other one-on-one time, that would be a bonus. I had to put all my eggs into that question.

We were being gathered for the greet. The families were set behind where the meet would happen, and the kids were seated around a large table. There were two director's chairs at the head of the table: one labeled "Tim Burton" and the other labeled "Artiste." Thinking that Tim would sit in his chair and Johnny would be in the other, I tried to sit as close as possible to the chair I guessed he'd be in. I ended up three chairs away from the "Artiste" chair.

Then … my life changed.

Tim walked in, right through the families. He looked exactly how he did in interviews on TV. Exactly how I imagined he would in person. I took a deep breath. This was happening. *Wait … If he was here … Then …* Johnny, as timid and shy as ever, walked a few paces behind Tim, and up to some of the family members. Tim made his way to the table and sat in the "Artiste" chair. That actually worked out perfectly, because based on who was in the other two chairs next to me, I did not have as clear a view of that one as I did the one Johnny sat in. Things *will* work out …

Johnny looked so nervous and fidgety. He took his seat, then looked around at us, and asked if anyone had taken any of the props. A little boy raised his hand, and Johnny said he was proud of him, and that he would have, too. *Wait, so I could have stolen something?* After that, he seemed more relaxed. He said he would get us all something before we left. After being encouraged by one of the "people in charge," he explained why he was dressed the way that he was (in makeup and costume). He explained a little about who Barnabas was, and why he was a cursed vampire, complete with long fingers (prosthetic extensions).

The Make-A-Wish people then called our names one at a time for us to ask our question to either Johnny, Tim, or the both of them. The other kids had some great questions. Some I already knew the answers to since I had read and seen almost every interview I could find throughout my eight years of fandom. It was still cool to hear Johnny say the answers in person, and he answered each with patience, as if it were the first time he'd ever been asked the question.

Again, I had planned to squeeze as much into my one question as I could, just in case this was the only time I was going to get to speak to Johnny. I had planned to start my question with "Happy International Talk like a Pirate Day." Boy, am I glad the person who went before me, went before me. Their entire question was "Did you know today is

International Talk like a Pirate Day?" I had no intention of stealing anyone's question, so I'm very glad they went first. Johnny said he'd never heard of the day before and began to speak like Captain Jack Sparrow. Hearing my favorite pirate speak like a pirate *on* Talk like a Pirate Day was the perfect cherry on top of the sundae.

Soon, I heard, "Our next question is from Katie." For a split second, I looked around, wondering if there was another Katie. *Right ... That's me.* I didn't know if there was another one and certainly didn't want to step on the toes of another wish kid (especially after I almost unintentionally stole someone's question).

By the time I realized I was *the* Katie, Johnny was staring at me. *His eyes!* I love his eyes. He can show so much expression through them, and they're so beautiful. I always wanted to be able to look into his eyes in person. (I knew he liked to hide behind sunglasses and was afraid he might be wearing some when I met him ... thankfully he wasn't.)

It was almost too much awesome with him looking me straight in the eye. In fact, there were a few times that he looked at me even when he was talking to other kids (probably because my entire body was bouncing up and down as I couldn't control my excitement). I kept having to break eye contact because I'm socially awkward, and I thought I would spontaneously combust if we held eye contact for too long.

After an embarrassingly awkward pause, I asked my question. A question I think came out eloquently, like all my interactions with Johnny, but who knows what that actually looked or sounded like from the outside. (My family confirmed later I didn't sound stupid.) I quickly wished him a happy Talk Like a Pirate Day, then asked how he takes his characters from the script to the screen, specifically what is his process from first reading the words to creating and getting into the character we see in the finished film. He said that was a good question and spent a decent amount of time thoughtfully answering it. He talked about getting flashes of what the character would be like, talking to the director to get their vision, trying different voices (maybe on his kids), taking bits of different inspiration throughout his life (like dogs and people), and putting it all together once he is in costume and makeup. The eye contact and listening to his voice ... if the world had ended at that moment, I don't think I could have been any more content.

When the Q and A session was over, Tim and Johnny were moved to the area where the camera was set up for the kids to get our photos taken. We had the option of taking a picture with Tim, Johnny, or both of them. We had to choose. I was not prepared for that choice! Tim went first, since he had to get back to filming as soon as possible. I really wanted evidence that I had met him. But I had always dreamed of a photo with just Johnny. The dilemma. *I suppose I could always crop Tim out of the group photo and then it would be just Johnny and me ... But that wouldn't be the same.* I asked someone to help me decide. Right before Tim left the photo area, one of the people in charge was so nice and let me sneak into two photos. They called Tim just in time before he left, and we quickly took a group picture.

I was SO CLOSE to Johnny! Have you ever been so close to something (or someone) you had dreamed about for much of your life? It's euphoric. My heart was beating out of my chest and I had to remind myself to breathe. Johnny put his hand on my shoulder. He was TOUCHING ME!!! And … that was consent to reciprocate, right? I tried to put my hand on his back. My brain wouldn't let me make contact at first. Like, I couldn't process he was right there. He was solid, and my hand would not go right through him like a ghost.

After the photo was taken (which I also didn't process … *Did I smile? Were my eyes open?*), Tim was told to get out (not by me), and the photographer took one of just Johnny and me. I barely processed that photo, but enough to ensure my eyes were open, and I was actually smiling. That sounds ridiculous … happiest moment of my life, one would assume I was smiling, no? I've been told (by several people) that I have a resting b*!@$ face. It's not that I'm not happy, but apparently I don't smile as much as other people. My face isn't designed to make smiling effortless. I have to consciously "check my face" and put a smile on for photos, even when I'm over-the-moon happy. In this case, I tried to make sure it wasn't a creepy smile. I was afraid I had a dumbstruck look due to how emotional I was. I may be my own worst critic, but this photo was going to be with me for the rest of my life. It had to be as wonderful as possible. And it was. I still use it as my computer desktop to this day (and it was my phone's lock screen for thirteen years … Until I got a selfie with Lana … And my phone background is a photo of Johnny and me from our next meet). As much as I do not like photos of myself, this one can immediately transport me back to how I felt that day and brings back wonderful memories of the whole experience.

I then had a private moment with just Johnny. He held my hand to comfort me as I poured my heart out. (But I didn't cry!) I told him what he has meant to me (as best as I could put into words in a few seconds as I hadn't rehearsed this). How he's the reason I'm here today. I even told him my insane dream to act with him one day. He said he'd be waiting for me, and I believed him … I still do.

Then, he hugged me. It was as if *he* didn't want to let go of *me*. Johnny gives the best hugs, and I would have been fine if he never let go.

When that phenomenal moment was over, I got my *Sweeney Todd* book for Tim to sign before he officially left. As I was asking him to sign it, I told him that it was my favorite movie … until that day when *Dark Shadows* was going to be my favorite. I'm sure that sounded quite silly. He was super polite and signed my book. I then waited for Johnny to be done with photos to get his autograph.

There was someone near me as we waited for Johnny's autograph who said they didn't have anything to get signed. That's exactly why I brought the blank paper. One of the volunteers asked if anyone had anything they could spare to get signed. I offered the paper. They asked if I would get it for them. I instinctively moved to go and get it. Then I realized that *Johnny Depp* was two feet away from me! I asked if they could retrieve it from my bag and told them where it was. As selfish as that seems, I was proud of myself for seizing my moment. I'm pretty quick to please others and often do things (like running to get paper for someone) at the expense of my own happiness. While that often is not a big deal, when one of my favorite people on the planet who is impossible to access is inches from me, I'm proud of myself for not giving up a second of that. The person who needed the paper still got it through my help, and I didn't give up a moment of being next to my hero. If I had stepped away, I would have lost my spot and likely would not have gotten Johnny's signature (at least not in my book that day). He was rushed back to work shortly after.

I handed Johnny my book when it was my turn. I didn't have my name tag on because I removed it for the photo (again, I planned to stare at it for the rest of my life and wanted it to be perfect), but he knew how to spell my name. Perhaps he looked at where Tim wrote it … But he still remembered it. He thought before he wrote and wrote the sweetest message.

As he was writing on someone else's item, he said he felt like Edward Scissorhands because of the finger extensions. That blew my mind, because he *was* Edward Scissorhands. One kid had the cover to the *Charlie and the Chocolate Factory* DVD signed. He said something in Willy Wonka's voice. These were little moments that kept reiterating to me, *this is Johnny Freaking Depp. Right here!*

Some of the kids started giving gifts to Johnny. One gave him two kangaroo dolls for his kids. One of his people tried to take them, and he acted like he wanted to keep them.

It was adorable. Without really thinking, I took the flying pig stone out of my pocket. I gave it to him and said that he had made my dream come true and that I hoped this brought him his dreams. He told me he would be the guardian of the pig, and if I ever wanted it back, I could come and get it from him. He then put it into his pocket and hugged me again.

He was then taken back to film, but he said he would be back. He was told that he wouldn't be able to return. I walked over to my family, and that is when I finally let my emotions boil over and I cried. I had met Johnny, and it was even better than I had dreamed it would be. Then, remembering that he had sat in the "Tim Burton" chair, I went over and sat down in it. I mean, how often can you say you sat in a chair after a famous person? Even though I wasn't the first person to do that since he had been there (my brother was), it was still cool.

I asked the property master to sign my book since he had worked on *Sweeney Todd* (and it will always be one of my favorites). Had I known who the photographer was, I would have liked him to sign the book as well.

After that unforgettable exchange, my family took a quick break while I lingered, soaking in the moment. My family used the bathroom before we left, while I waited. We were soon being escorted out because the wish was over. I could have stayed there forever. The people in charge had gift bags for all the kids and their siblings, and someone came with a plate of finger extensions Johnny had used in the filming of the movie he wanted us to have. Each kid was given two finger extensions. That was awesome. Not only were they used in the movie, but Johnny had directly had them attached to his hands. As I was waiting for my family to be done in the bathroom, I could see on the monitor that Johnny was already back to filming. I burned the moments he was filming into my memory, because there was a good chance my pig stone was still in his pocket, and it's a moment I felt close to my hero.

With the wish officially over, we said our goodbyes and headed back to the hotel, still buzzing from everything we had experienced. We were driven back to our hotel and had the remainder of the trip to explore the city. That day, the package with the itinerary finally arrived at the hotel. Better late than never, right? And the remaining days we enjoyed ordering off the menu at breakfast since we learned that was included. We got to try some interesting British breakfasts.

An unforeseen benefit of going to London was I had the opportunity to see one of Johnny's films that was never released in America. It's called *The Brave*, and he wrote, directed, and starred in it. I had purchased the DVD a few years before, back when I didn't understand about how DVDs have regions for different countries. I just thought if I found a copy, I would be able to watch it. When I put it into my American DVD player, it told me that I was unable to watch that region. That's when the internet explained to me how it was feasible to keep a film out of a country. But … London was in the region of the DVD I owned … AND … there was a DVD player in our hotel room. So, I got to watch one of his films that had escaped my reach for eight years. It's a powerful movie. I'm very happy I got to see it, especially on a trip as special as my wish. I later purchased a portable Region 2 DVD player, so I can watch it whenever I want.

We had two more full days in London, then a few hours on the final day before we were picked up to return to the airport. In this time, we explored as much as we could with our limited knowledge of the city and culture. We did a hop-on, hop-off bus tour (like most tourists on short trips do), as this was something that would get us around to the major sights of the city, would teach us about these locations through the audio tour, and was a place to sit if we needed to rest while we were out.

We got to see the Science Museum, which was great because I love science (says the Chemistry teacher). We saw many of the tourist locations such as the Tower of London, Tower Bridge, London Bridge, the London Eye, Piccadilly Circus, Big Ben and Parliament, Hamleys, Harrods … the works. We didn't have time to *do* everything, but we did get to walk around a lot. My brother and I explored Whitechapel at night (because Johnny did a film on Jack the Ripper called *From Hell*), and we tried to get to Saint Paul Cathedral at night. I'm not going to go into detail on why we didn't get there … You can ask my brother. Let's just say, I learned about some of my GI issues through the experience.

The last full day we were in London, Make-A-Wish sent us to Madame Tussauds Wax Museum. That was a cool bonus, where we learned about the process of how the wax statues are made and got to see the celebrities made out of wax. My favorite, of course, was Captain Jack Sparrow, who was staged on an area that looked like a ship. Sometimes the statue is dressed like Johnny, and other times, Jack. This was also a photo opportunity, and we were given a free photo with our ticket. This was a picture with "Johnny" I was able to go home with from my wish trip. The real one I had to call and ask for after *Dark Shadows* came out. I was actually in London when I called because I returned the following summer to study abroad.

The morning of the day we were to return home, D.J. and I walked the areas around our hotel with Thumper. As we took final pictures in front of the Tower of London and Tower Bridge, it was impossible to not reflect on the incredible trip that was coming to an end. It seemed like a dream. A week prior, I was being told that my wish to meet Johnny was going to be granted. And now, my family had traveled to another country to meet the man of my dreams. And it had been perfect.

My wish made me fall in love with London, and I decided that studying abroad would be a wonderful excuse to return. I only had one final summer in order to do so as I was a junior and every remaining semester was already spoken for in terms of what courses I had to take. I justified doing a summer to cover my final honors program course (which I had previously abandoned the idea of, because I didn't have time for all the requirements in my regular schedule).

Our return home was thankfully uneventful. Everything was on time, the food on the flight was delicious, and we were delivered safely home from our trip among the stars.

We were greeted at home by a message on our answering machine—unfortunately, I had missed an opportunity to be in a movie with some famous actors. I'd auditioned shortly before we left and got the call while we were away. I called back, but they had already moved past that scene and couldn't use me anymore. *Oh, well*—it just wasn't meant to be. I would take my experience with Johnny and Tim in London every single time over being an extra in some other film. My wish experience did encourage me to keep going out for background roles (after all, Johnny said he would be waiting for me …). I started getting a few, which is much more difficult than you would expect (maybe a little bit because I live in an area that doesn't make as many movies as Hollywood or London).

When we returned to reality, I didn't come down from cloud nine for several months. I mentioned that I had met Johnny Depp to everyone I talked to. I couldn't stop smiling.

Some of my long-term side effects were even beginning to get better.

I was happier.

I was no longer as crippled by survivor's guilt. Instead, that was replaced with a voice that said I should find a way to give back to Make-A-Wish. It took me two years to set up my first fundraiser and one more year before I became a wish granter. More on *all* that later.

I met Johnny once I regained a good amount of my health and strength—four years after my diagnosis. It was one of the happiest moments of my life, and I'm sure it will remain so for a long time. Standing in his presence and telling him what he meant to me exceeded every dream I'd had (simply the fact I was able to coherently communicate with him was a huge win).

That day, I fell in love all over again, and I'll hold those memories close forever. Somehow, I had a feeling this wasn't the last time I'd see him. After all, my goal was still to work with him one day—specifically, to act alongside him (and while we're ~~being delulu~~ ... *dreaming big* ... let's add Lana Parrilla too). Technically, I've "worked" with Johnny already, but—that's also a story for later.

Chapter 5
Tutoring

Because I was in and out of the hospital, returning to regular school wasn't possible. To keep up with my classmates and stay on schedule for senior year, I had to begin homebound tutoring. I've always loved school. I was your typical "teacher's pet" who never missed a day if I could help it. Being told I would not be going back to school was killing me and nearly drove me insane.

Education, and extracurricular activities (mainly the Drama Club), were my life. My priorities were about grades and staying on track for college. I was in the highest level of classes being offered, constantly challenging myself however I could, and I was currently struggling my way through my first college-level class (Biology). I say "struggling" because school never came easy to me, but I always enjoyed pushing myself to the next level. Reading, writing, and learning new material have always been things I've had to work tirelessly at. While I was ranked fairly high in my class when I was diagnosed (not that that matters, but it *did* to my teenage self as a personal drive to keep working to improve myself ... Plus, I had an older brother, and everything is a competition with siblings), I would not describe myself as "smart." Instead, I would say that I am "determined" and "dedicated" (aka … "stubborn"). In the end, these were invaluable skills which helped get me through everything.

When you're not able to attend school where I live, you're entitled to homebound tutoring to continue your education. For some reason, this was a feat to get set up and started. It almost seemed as if someone wanted me to stay back and repeat the eleventh grade. While that is a perfectly good option for some people … I was *not* one of them. I had a plan for my life. Clearly that plan needed adjustment (after adjustment …), but being told by an unknown authority that it would be "easier" if I just repeated a grade … easier on *whom*? First of all, I had *completed* more than 25% of the year before I was diagnosed. Sure, that's not a lot, but that's 25% more than I was willing to redo for no good reason. And to me, with the type of person I was, giving in to repeating the grade would have been admitting something I wasn't willing to concede to. Secondly, that would mean an extra year of what precious time I may have had left spent in school. While I do love it, just not quite *that* much. Thirdly, I already had a class ring that said "2009." (I officially dated myself there.) I was going to graduate in 2009 … if I was there to see it. Fourthly … (there were a few reasons), AP Chemistry was going to be offered the next year. There was no guarantee that it would be offered the following year (which it wasn't, but it did come back eventually). I had to be ready to take the course, which meant being finished with my current classes. Fifthly, it was something to focus on to get my mind off things. I'm sure there are more reasons that guided my steadfastness to my decision, but those are the main ones. And isn't five enough?

Despite the obstacles to getting tutoring started, one unexpected act of kindness helped move things forward. I owe tutoring getting off the ground a few months in to my Chemistry teacher. He was the first one who stepped up to offer to be one of my tutors. I emailed him while I was in the hospital toward the beginning of treatment and went to visit the school as soon as I got out. Visiting was nice, and I never wanted that feeling to end (like nothing had changed … even though everything had). At the same time, I also suddenly felt like an outsider in my own school. I knew I wasn't going to be finishing my junior year the way I had planned, and that the "best-year-of-my-life," senior year, had a huge question mark over its head.

That was the day he offered to be one of my tutors. That took a lot of pressure off and meant so much. At that point, I assumed tutors would be people I'd never met before. I didn't realize they would be teachers I already knew. In fact, that subject (Biology) became the one that kept me focused and on track.

When everything was underway, I had tutoring for each course once a week (when I was out of the hospital) at my town's local library. Libraries are the best. The smell of brand new and well-loved books greeting you when you enter the automatic front doors to the building … We would often get there before my tutors since we didn't have much else to do. We would wait in the purply plush armchairs in the reading area.

Some weeks, tutoring was the only time I got out of the house (aside from trips to CCMC, which half the time ended in being admitted).

Once tutoring sessions were in progress, I quickly realized how difficult learning had become. I was suffering from what's commonly called "chemo brain." My short-term memory, especially the first months of treatment, was awful. I would forget mid-sentence what I was talking about. This was a side effect of the chemotherapy, which is why it earned the name "chemo brain" (also known as "chemo fog"). God bless my tutors for their patience with me.

I remember the tutoring sessions themselves more than any content we covered. Although, I do remember getting to write a research paper on Johnny Depp (one of the *numerous* times throughout my education I was able to work him into my assignments). These sessions allowed me to be myself. In a class full of other students, I struggled with what others thought of me (I've tried my whole life to "not care," but once your confidence is damaged, it can be difficult to fix). I ask *a lot* of questions. One, because I'm confused easily and want to get clarification. Two, I'm extremely curious and want to learn as much as I can. I'm not sure if you were the type of student growing up who asked questions or the type who didn't like the kid who spoke in class frequently. But I felt pressure to not speak up in class as often as I wanted to. That was not an issue when it was one-on-one. I felt free to ask or say anything relevant.

Those tutoring sessions didn't just help me keep up with school—they helped shape the kind of teacher I wanted to become. I had already decided I wanted to be a teacher, but seeing what an impact you can have on a student further validated my decision. I'm grateful for each of the incredible educators who stepped up to help me get through my junior year. I'm sure I was a nuisance, but the time they put in really made a difference. I would not have been able to graduate on time if not for them (and timing was critical down the line for many other events I would have missed if I was a year behind in my education).

Later, when I finally became a teacher myself, I carried those lessons—and the gratitude—with me into the classroom. But stepping into that new role brought its own kind of identity shift.

I went from being the "cancer girl" at college (okay, I wasn't *called* that, but everyone knew) to a blank slate when I was hired at my full-time job. I didn't tell anyone at my current place of employment, or my students, for the first year or so. I wanted to be "normal." It was a fresh start where no one knew me for once (that was odd, and liberating). For the first time since I had been diagnosed, I was not being defined by cancer.

But things or comments crop up, and it becomes difficult to explain if people don't know. Like, if I mentioned a random side effect (such as I can't open water bottles because of the lack of strength in my fingers), a concern (like, maybe a random chest pain was something to worry about, even in my twenties), or meeting Johnny Depp (because that is really difficult to *not* talk about … I consider myself as having a good filter if I have ever had a conversation with you and NOT brought it up).

Over time, I started to connect with some students if I knew they were battling their own health crisis, or if they had a family member dealing with cancer. That would give me the opening to say, *"I may not understand exactly what you're going through, but I'm a cancer survivor and I'm here if you want to talk."* Maybe I didn't tell anyone at first because a small, irrational part of me worried that someone might question whether I deserved to have survived. Or worse … wish I hadn't. I know that sounds dramatic, but survivor's guilt has a way of warping even the most logical thoughts. That sounds stupid out loud … on paper … (because children are all wonderful and would *never* wish that about their teacher …), but I didn't want to jinx anything. Yes, all kids, especially my students, are wonderful. But why risk it?

I'll never be risk-free of a secondary cancer … One I might not survive, especially because of the tolerance I've built up to the medicines already used on me. I'm a member of a parish, and there were several people praying for me and my family throughout my journey. I believe in the power of prayer and do think it helped in my survival.

I teach the same grade and age I was when I left school to battle cancer. It's interesting, to basically be in a perpetual loop of the year I missed. But obviously I'm an adult with life experiences, and times are quite different than back in 2007.

Every day I see kids think that some little aspect of their life is the end of the world, when in reality, many of what bothers your average teenager doesn't matter to the extent you think it does while in the moment. (I'm not saying that their lives are easy or that *nothing* is important; some children's lives are much harder than others.) It frustrates me when otherwise healthy kids that have every opportunity available to them are doing things like skipping class or making other developmentally appropriate silly decisions I didn't have the chance to make (not that I *would* have … but that's not the point). I want the best for each of my students and hope they discover what truly matters in life—before they have to face something that forces them to.

Chapter 6
True Colors

The number of people who told my family, "Let us know if you need anything," was truly heartwarming. We were overwhelmed with the massive changes to our lives and didn't want to burden anyone by asking for help, so we mostly didn't. But that didn't stop people from offering assistance in every way they could. It was incredible how our community came together to support my family throughout my treatment.

An organization my mom had been involved with for years—one that my brother and I are now also members of—organized a town-wide pancake breakfast fundraiser to help with medical expenses. Seeing who showed up, who bought tickets even if they couldn't attend, and even strangers who wanted to support us, blew us away. It was an amazing experience, and I'm so honored that the people who organized it cared so deeply about my family to put in all that effort. I can't thank them, or everyone who helped make the event such a success, enough.

It would have been wonderful if I was feeling better the day of the breakfast, but you take the wins where you can.

That morning, every bone and joint in my body ached so badly it brought me to tears. All I could think was, *something must be terribly wrong.* That shadow in the back of my mind—*Is this a secondary cancer? Is my cancer back? Is this it?*—was screaming louder than ever. I ended up back in the hospital soon after, but thankfully everything was as okay as could be expected, nowhere near as bad as my imagination feared.

It felt like everyone in my school sent me a card at some point. Every club I was part of sent messages to cheer me up and remind me they were thinking about me. I loved reading each one. I also became pen pals with two girls in my class who sent me actual letters in the mail—remember sending handwritten letters? It was a wonderful connection to those amazing young women, and their letters always lifted my spirits.

My Spanish teacher even had the entire class sign a card for me every month for the rest of the school year. That meant so much. It's one thing to hear, "Oh, someone is sick … too bad," and move on. It's another to keep reminding that person they're still thought of throughout their battle.

When people want to show they care, they often bring or send gifts. I've always been awkward about accepting handouts, so I'm sure I looked like, *Why would you give me this toy or book when some other kid could use it more?* Even if I didn't say it, my confused and dumbfounded expression probably said it all. I'll never forget when family friends— those special "aunts and uncles" with no real blood relation—gave me a Nintendo DS and games. That was my first handheld video game system since the Game Boy Advance (which, by the way, was a Christmas gift from Santa). This was incredible because, back then, cell phones didn't really have games … at least not the flip phone I had. Am I dating myself again? (Kids, ask your parents what a flip phone is—though they're kind of making a comeback.)

Diagnosed in the middle of November, we found ourselves moving in and out of the hospital as Christmas approached. Thankfully, I was discharged just in time to spend the holiday at home—something I was absolutely determined to do. My family had made plans months before my diagnosis to visit my uncle (a "real" uncle, not one of those honorary ones) in Oklahoma for Christmas, but I wasn't having it. Any other time of year, sure—no problem. But Christmas? That had to be spent at home. Around my tree, with my immediate family and our traditions. And, lucky me, I got my way. I'll never forget coming home on Christmas Eve to find that my brother and dad had put up the tree as a surprise. Until that moment, none of us really felt much like celebrating, but that sight changed everything.

Around the holidays, various toy drives pop up for kids who are stuck in the hospital. Even though there's almost always some small gifts or toys meant to spark joy for those undergoing treatment, there's a bigger movement to make sure children who aren't well have a happy holiday season. At the time, I still hadn't quite accepted that I was "one of those sick kids," so accepting gifts from those drives felt a little wrong. I've always been someone who gives—donating toys to children in need whenever I can—but being on the receiving end of that generosity was harder than I expected.

Emotionally, I was all over the place—and it wasn't just the guilt about accepting kindness. My body and mind were changing in ways I couldn't quite understand or control. Chemotherapy changes the chemical balance of your body, altering how you feel and how you behave. It made me incredibly emotional. I found myself crying at the cheesiest commercials, then instantly snapping if the cafeteria ran out of soft pretzels (but seriously, who wouldn't get upset about that?). No matter how much I tried to keep calm, these emotions felt like they weren't entirely mine—they bubbled up unexpectedly and without warning. On top of that, remember I was put on birth control to stop my menstrual cycle, which basically shoved me into a mini menopause and only added to the mood swings.

I met people who really understood these changes happening to me, and others who didn't quite get it. As difficult as it must have been to tolerate my mood swings, I was lucky to have some amazing people around who knew which parts I could control—and which parts I couldn't— and never held those struggles against me.

For the people who did take it personally, all I can say is this: "I'm sorry."

But emotions and misunderstandings weren't the only hurdles I faced. As time went on, another reality became clear—how people respond when they think they can relate to your experience even when they really can't.

The funny thing about going through any kind of trauma or ordeal is that you'll inevitably meet people who want to relate to you—no matter what. You could be the very first person to experience something, and others will still insist they know exactly what you're feeling because they've had a "similar" experience. But their version rarely even comes close to what you're going through. Whenever I tried to talk about something troubling me—or, heaven forbid, just vent—people felt the need to jump in with advice on how *they* handled their problems.

I have to admit, since becoming a teacher, I've caught myself doing this sometimes. But I like to think there's a small difference: when a student opens up to me about something I can't relate to, I listen—full stop. If I *do* have a relatable experience, I share it only if the student seems open to hearing it. And if I want to give advice but can't directly relate, I tell them that upfront.

I encountered plenty of well-meaning people sharing their stories. Wonderful people, truly—please don't misunderstand me. But as heartfelt as their intentions were, their stories didn't ease my pain. On the contrary, they reminded me of how isolated cancer made me feel, how far removed my life had become from "normal" experiences. Even though cancer is common, each person's journey is unique. I always knew there were people who had it worse than I did, but I still had to cope with *my* path.

This is a big reason I never went to therapy at the time— even though I definitely should have. I thought it would be like talking to someone who couldn't truly relate. I needed people who could just listen when I needed to talk without trying to give answers or advice that felt unhelpful (which … isn't that what therapy should be?). When I wanted to talk about how an intramuscular injection had severed a nerve in my leg, I didn't want to hear about someone stubbing their toe. When I needed to vent about no longer being able to climb stairs because my muscles were too weak, the last thing I needed was someone comparing it to their headache (which I have too many of my own experiences with). I wasn't trying to be unempathetic, but everyone has moments when things need to be about them.

If you ever find yourself caring for a loved one with cancer, please try to listen. You likely won't be able to solve all their problems, and no amount of kind words can cure their cancer. Just listen. Care. Empathize. Be there. And remember to take care of yourself along the way.

I found the best listeners in the most unexpected places. One was a teacher—without whom I don't know how I would've made it through. (Did you guess it was my Chemistry teacher?) He was there for me to vent to, and actually had useful life experiences (unfortunately). But he never pushed his stories on me or dismissed what I was going through. He listened whenever I needed to talk and never told me it was a bad time or that he didn't want to hear it. He was more than I could've asked for, and certainly more than I deserved. Looking back, I feel a little guilty for how comfortable I felt opening up to him—not that I regret having him as a confidant, but for any awkward conversations I dragged him into. He didn't ask for it—I just somehow felt completely safe and at ease talking to him.

Not every teacher is that exceptional, but every child deserves at least one educator they can trust like that, if needed. I aspire to be that for any of my students who could use it.

On the flip side, I was lucky to have an incredible friend who had a similar experience a few years before me. She was always there to support me, cheer me on, and lovingly tell me to suck it up when I was whining about something trivial. I truly needed that—and still do. She reminded me, even at my lowest points, how fortunate I was, how much worse things could have been, and how important it was to focus on the positives. I try really hard, and I hope she'd be proud of where I am today. Granted, this book includes *a lot* of complaining (previous drafts included even *more*), but that was part of processing my journey. If anyone in a similar situation can take even one positive thing from my story, then this book was worth writing. But more on her later.

Throughout the entire process, I also learned what friendship truly means. Friends I'd been close to my whole life reacted to my illness in ways I never could have imagined. I'll never forget the look of terror on one friend's face when they literally recoiled from me, as if I had the plague. It was like being in the same room suddenly felt too close for comfort—like they might catch leukemia just from touching me. To be fair, I had heard rumors going around school that cancer was contagious … which, spoiler alert, it is *not*! Still, we were in high school, and that made it no less shocking.

I still love this friend, and I understand that cancer is terrifying for everyone involved. But that moment stayed with me, a reminder of how isolated I felt—even when my friends were physically right there.

Overall, my friends were exactly what you'd hope for in a support system, and I'm so thankful for each one. They stayed by my side, visited me, brought movies (physical DVDs were still a big thing back then), and kept me updated on the life I'd temporarily left behind. I'll always treasure their kindness, and that of their families, during my time away from school.

When I returned for my senior year, I expected things to pick up where they left off. Of course, that was impossible. I had missed nearly three-quarters of a year—months of shared memories, experiences, and normal teenage life. Junior year is huge. I hadn't even taken the SATs, looked at universities, or applied anywhere. All of that had to be crammed into the fall of my senior year, while my friends were already receiving their acceptance letters. I felt like our group's dynamic had shifted, and looking back, that makes sense. They had kept growing together, planning their futures, while I was grappling with the very real uncertainty of whether I'd even have a tomorrow.

I'd imagined senior year would be the greatest year of my life—or at least that was the plan before I became the "cancer kid." It's supposed to be your swan song, the year you finally get to be "top dog" at school. Even though, honestly, I never felt that way. What special powers does being a senior really give you? That said, getting older is an accomplishment and absolutely worth celebrating—just not something that makes you better than anyone younger.

Instead, senior year was nothing like I had planned.

It started that summer when I went to have my senior portraits taken. I felt terrible that day and looked like the walking dead—paler than this page is. We didn't realize it then, but (we really should have guessed) I needed a blood transfusion and was about to check into the hospital. That was one of the few times I wore my wig. It wasn't very comfortable—it had to be taped to my scalp, which felt like it was perpetually sunburned.

I'll never forget the day I was measured for the wig. The people helping me were kind and patient, but I was in a terrible mood because everything hurt that day. Some days brought sudden, inexplicable pain, and that was one of them. I was also struggling emotionally with the uncertainty of whether I'd ever have my own hair again. The measuring process involved placing and moving tape on my scalp, which burned terribly because my skin was so sensitive. I felt awful for not being more grateful to those who helped me—definitely not my best day. If I could go back, I'd handle it differently.

When the senior photos came back, I hated looking at them. I looked sick, and I told my parents (though I doubt they would have listened because they seemed to like the pictures) not to use them in my obituary if I died. I didn't want everyone to see me like that—especially not as the last image of me. I wanted a nice photo, one taken back when I was healthy.

Returning to school after such a long absence was a shock. Nothing felt the same. Starting the fall as a "regular" student again was … odd. I had changed so much in the ten months I'd been away. I'd been forced to mature in ways teenagers shouldn't have to.

To help me manage school safely and keep up as best as I could, several accommodations were put in place. I was allowed to visit the nurse whenever I needed, use the elevator (since I still couldn't climb stairs—even just a few to get on the bus), and have alternative transportation instead of the bus (again, because stairs were impossible). I had antibacterial wipes to sanitize my desk before class (because germs were dangerous to my weakened immune system), permission to leave class early to avoid crowds, permission to keep my cell phone with me in case I needed help or if I fell (this was before kids having phones in school became normal), and more.

My senior year ended up being the one I missed the most days of school (if you don't count junior year, when I stopped going to the building altogether). I missed days for treatments, clinic visits, or simply because I wasn't well enough. My blood counts were always low, and my immune system suppressed. Whenever I was around others, I diligently watched for sneezes, sniffles, or coughs. Catching anything could have been life-threatening. I social distanced and carried hand sanitizer everywhere. Honestly, I was way ahead of the curve for the COVID pandemic!

I was only enrolled in about four classes that year, while the norm was six or seven. I usually took as many classes as possible, but that year, I took only what I had to—plus AP Chemistry.

I had to drop from advanced placement courses to regular honors classes. At my school, AP classes were basically university-level courses, while honors were still challenging but more manageable. I'd been used to pushing myself hard in AP classes, so honors felt easier by comparison.

I remember my Calculus class especially well—I had extra time after finishing work to focus on how the teacher taught. She was fantastic and even answered some of my "teacher" questions, since I was planning to become an educator myself. That made the class extra productive for me, and I'm grateful—when I took Calculus in college, despite my short-term memory issues, I was able to rely on my notes from that class to help me succeed.

I was also in a creative writing class where I worked on the early form of *Thumper's Adventures* and wrote my first short memoir, which later became my college essay. So … pretty helpful!

AP Chemistry was the class that really required my time and brainpower. Since it was the only class demanding that much focus, I was able to give it the effort it needed despite my finite energy. At the end of the year, I did very well on the AP exam, which I was proud of—especially given my memory challenges.

At my school back then, your gym class was paired with your science class because of the way the schedule worked. So, your gym classmates were usually the same as your science classmates.

My gym class that year was wonderful! I never questioned whether we did the usual curriculum or if our gym teacher was less intense with us because we were the "nerds" in AP Chemistry. Either way, it was awesome. Technically, I was excused from gym, but I ended up fully participating most days, when I felt well enough. My teacher even commented once that I didn't have to, but I was more into it than some of the others in the class.

We did a lot of fun things that year—yard games like bocce and croquet, and we played pickleball and badminton. Those last two were a bit more physically challenging with my limitations but still enjoyable. Basically, as long as I reminded my body not to run (or I'd fall) and didn't swing my arms too quickly (since I couldn't reach over my head), it was a great time.

Even in moments like those, where I could laugh and participate, the reality of my illness was never far from my mind.

I get that it can be really hard to talk to someone who's sick, especially when you don't know what to say or even if they'll get better. It's tricky to always find the right words— we're all human, after all. But some of the things said to me still caught me off guard.

I'll never forget telling someone about my Make-A-Wish experience. After I shared, they paused, their face went blank, and they asked if I was currently dying. If you're one of the people who thinks Make-A-Wish is only for kids who are terminal, that's not true. It's for children facing critical illnesses. Many kids who get wishes go on to live long, full lives.

But there was another common reaction I encountered—something that happened even more often than that awkward Make-A-Wish moment. People would tell me how lucky I was. At the time, and even now, that always struck me as a strange thing to say. Sure, I was fortunate in many ways—I survived, I had support, I found strength I never knew I had. But *lucky*? *Lucky to get cancer? To spend endless days in the hospital? To miss out on the normal milestones and freedoms my peers enjoyed? To face the terrifying reality that I might not live to see adulthood? To endure the trauma that comes with all of that?* No, I don't think I was lucky at all.

Some would say things like, "You're so lucky you don't have to run the mile," as if dodging a dreaded gym test was some kind of prize. For years, I was always the slowest runner—being last every year wasn't exactly a victory. If anyone had wanted to trade places with me, I would have gladly taken the mile run over the needles shoved into my spine and hip every other week.

Becoming the "sick kid" changed how people saw me, and their true colors showed through—good, bad, and indifferent. Some were incredibly kind and supportive to me and my family. Others seemed terrified or, oddly, even jealous of my situation. But through it all, I witnessed how much genuine goodness there is in people—a reality that often gets lost in the noise of the world. That was a comforting, even hopeful, thing to discover firsthand.

PART THREE

The Emotional Lessons and Reflections

Chapter 7
Life and Loss

It truly is better to have loved and lost than never to have loved at all. But it's still better never to have lost in the first place.

I had the incredible privilege of growing close to some truly remarkable survivors who were battling the same cancer I was. The first, a young woman around my age, was diagnosed just a month after me. From the very beginning, she became a trusted confidant—a lifeline as we navigated the uncharted waters of this terrifying new reality. We shared some fears, frustrations, and the small victories as we tried to make sense of this "new normal" that had suddenly taken over our lives. Having someone who understood the physical and emotional challenges firsthand made all the difference. We leaned on each other, finding strength in our shared experience, even on the days when it felt like the weight of it all might crush us.

Another survivor I met had recently finished her treatment. She was nothing short of extraordinary—a steadfast rock of confidence and unwavering support. Whenever I felt overwhelmed or unsure, she was there to steady me, to remind me of my own resilience. She immediately took me under her wing. At times when I found myself sinking into despair or complaining about the side effects, she would gently but firmly give me a much-needed kick in the pants. She'd remind me that no matter what I was going through, I was still standing. Even though her treatment was over, she was bravely facing the long-term side effects of chemotherapy and a bone marrow transplant, but never once did I hear her complain. Instead, she focused on hope, healing, and the strength we all had inside.

One evening remains etched in my memory. My town's Relay for Life was hosting a fundraiser at a local restaurant, but I was in college with no way to get there on my own. Without hesitation, she picked me up from campus, drove us to the event, and despite my repeated attempts to pay for our meal, refused to accept a single penny. After we ate, she drove me back to school. That night we shared not only a delicious meal but also precious moments of connection and understanding that transcended words. She went out of her way to make sure I was part of something bigger, reminding me that we were never alone in this fight.

That evening was the second to last time I saw her.

The final time we met, I asked her a question that may have seemed strange, but that's one of my quirks: "What do you want to be when you grow up?" Not because she wasn't already an adult, but because I've always believed it's never too late to dream, to chase something beyond the present moment. Her answer was simple yet profound: she didn't know *yet*.

I admired her deeply—her strength, her humility, and her enduring spirit. She was beloved by everyone who knew her, a pillar of the largest volunteer organization in our town. She was so nurturing and respected that everyone affectionately called her "Ma." When I received the call that she was seriously ill, I felt a hollow ache in my chest. She wanted me to know, to prepare for what was coming. And then, shortly after, the devastating news that she had passed. The turnout at her funeral was staggering—a standing-room-only service with a line stretching out the door. It was like something out of a movie, a powerful testament to how many lives she had touched. The sheer volume of people mourning her loss made it clear: she was deeply loved and would be severely missed.

Her life was a shining example of how one person truly can make a difference in the world. She left a permanent mark on everyone she met, and her legacy continues to inspire. I am so grateful to have known her—to have witnessed firsthand the ripple effect of kindness, courage, and compassion.

But alongside the comfort and strength she gave me came the sharp, unrelenting reality of loss. Through her, I learned that even in the face of death, love endures. And that memory, that love, can carry us through the darkest of times.

Concurrently, I found a similar bond with another incredible young woman named Cindy. I am so thankful for the brief time I had as her friend. Though our paths crossed in the hospital under unfortunate circumstances, we quickly connected over shared experiences and small things—like our matching fuzzy slippers.

I honestly do not remember how we connected. I didn't get out of my hospital room much, which didn't make for the best mingling environment. My parents did get out of the room (as they should have) and have always been keener on striking up a conversation with someone than I ever will be. (They are the type of people who can spend five minutes with a stranger and know everything there is to know about them. I'm the type of person who can spend an hour with someone and can't answer a question as simple as "what's their last name?") Perhaps they met Cindy's parents and got to know one another in the kitchen or common room. They probably discovered that we were both having a difficult time and could be someone for the other to talk to. That is likely the scenario. I have the idea in my head that coffee or breakfast was involved. But this was a part of life at the hospital I wasn't involved with: the family area to hang out and get away from the rooms for a moment. A place to maybe pretend for one second that your child wasn't in the other room fighting for their life as you are struggling to keep it together for them. A place to maybe cry for a minute when the weight of the world was crushing everything down on top of you. A place to find other people going through similar unspeakably horrible trials, and either find a shoulder to lean on or wisdom to be shared. Or maybe, just a place to grab a cup of coffee, the occasionally donated baked good refreshment, or a Popsicle from the freezer.

Any way that it happened, I remember I started to visit Cindy in her room. Psychologically, we were in a similar place. Physically, we had different cancers that were trying to kill us, one of which succeeded. Cindy was bravely fighting a brain tumor. I remember walking in wearing my purple fuzzy slippers (which I wore everywhere around the hospital). Cindy used to have a pair like mine in pink, and this was a silly thing we bonded over. Pink and purple had been my favorite colors growing up … They still are.

My IV pole and I walked down to her room a few times while we were both in the hospital together. I forgot who got to leave first. It was probably me, because I had the luxury of getting pretty regular vacations from the hospital where I got to go to the luxurious resort of my house. With my *own* bed. With non-cafeteria-food cuisine (the cafeteria workers were all a delight, but any food can get tiring day after day). There were a few other times I bumped into either Cindy or her mom around the hospital after that stay. I visited her once when I was there for an outpatient treatment. Then some time went by, and I lost the ability to connect with her since I didn't know her last name (told you I was bad at that … Plus, this was before everyone was connected through the internet and cell phones 24/7). That doesn't mean I stopped thinking about her or her family, or hoping she would be okay.

At college, I became involved in an organization that supported the oncology clinic at CCMC and gave a scholarship to a patient being treated there. I had the honor of receiving several similar scholarships, which was one of the reasons I wanted to pay it forward to other patients.

At some point, we received a newsletter from CCMC. In one of the photos, I recognized Cindy. She looked good, and it was a fairly recent image. That made me very happy. To add to that, under the photo was her full name! I had one of those bad feelings in the pit of my stomach, for no reason I could put my finger on. Later that night, when I got to my laptop in my dorm room (again, we didn't have the internet in our pockets … Or at least I didn't yet), I looked her up. A part of me was hoping to find her Facebook page and send her a friend request (kids, you can ask your parents what that is later).

Instead, I found what I was dreading. An obituary for my first similarly aged friend.

I read through burning tears as I struggled to find the air to fill my lungs. Cindy had passed away after a two-and-a-half-year battle with cancer, was an incredible person, and everyone who knew her was left to learn how to keep moving forward without her in their lives. She passed away one month to the day I was about to finish my treatment. A treatment that was scheduled to last exactly how long her battle lasted.

Losing Cindy was devastating. Her passing marked the beginning of a complicated and heavy feeling that would stay with me long after my own treatment ended. This was the beginning of my bout with survivor's guilt. I say "bout" as if it's 100% over. Through a lot of time and figuring everything out, it has gotten better (to the point where it doesn't cripple me), but I can be triggered into these emotions again. Like, I would be lying if I said writing about Cindy (or any of the other people lost) in this book didn't bring up some of these feelings and tears. But I'm in such a better place than I was years ago.

If you've never heard of it, survivor's guilt is a *wonderful* (insert sarcasm font when it's invented) feeling that can develop in people who have survived a life-threatening event or situation. They can feel guilty for various reasons. The one I experienced was because they/we survived while others did/do not. There was a very brief time when I was first diagnosed that I asked *"why me?"* from a selfish point of view, as in, why did I have to get sick? That quickly changed to a different form of *"why me?"* At that point, why was I surviving while others weren't? It didn't, and *still* doesn't, make any sense. Kids who had the same diagnosis as me, and were doing everything right, were passing away. Kids who had other cancers, like Cindy, were passing away. Other people who were fighting just as hard as I was, were passing away.

Why was I alive?

That question sent me down a gloomy rabbit hole. I started to have really dark opinions about myself, that I didn't deserve to survive (not that I was going to do anything to change that, but it fed into the guilt that I wasn't worthy of surviving over any other person). I was guilty just for the fact that I was alive.

This, like many emotions, isn't something you can simply "get over" or "let it go." Looking back, I should have found a more focused support group or went to counseling to deal with my feelings. But in the thick of it, I knew it sounded odd for thinking my survival was in any way tied to others. I also didn't know where to even start looking for the right support for that. And even if I did, I thought I would sound stupid talking to someone about how I felt bad for surviving. I just put my head down, cried a lot to myself, talked to my close support circle, and focused on staying alive (continuing to fight for my own life).

I do not recommend doing this on your own.

Once I was medically "out of the woods," I realized professional help could have made a difference. If you or someone you know struggles with survivor's guilt or mental health challenges, it's okay—more than okay—to ask for help.

My Make-A-Wish experience was life-changing for several reasons. In terms of my ongoing struggle with survivor's guilt, it became an epiphany. It taught me something I now hold on to tightly: we all have a purpose. Each of us has a choice—to make the world brighter, or not.

I realized that I had been given a second chance at life, and I needed to use it. Doing good became my answer. Shortly after my own wish was granted, I threw myself into volunteering for Make-A-Wish and supporting initiatives connected to children's cancer research and hospitals. (It's why a portion of the proceeds of this book goes directly to those causes.)

Looking back, I was one of the lucky ones. Nearly every night, someone stayed with me at the hospital. My family always came up to eat dinner with me.

That's when I began to truly understand how fortunate I was. Some children's parents had to work constantly just to keep food on the table or cover the mountain of medical bills. Between my parents' work schedules and my brother's law school commitments, someone was still always there overnight to keep me company.

I also saw children who didn't even have a proper diagnosis. They were moved from doctor to doctor, test to test, without any clear answers. Without a diagnosis, effective treatment is almost impossible. Even with a diagnosis, treatment doesn't necessarily mean a cure.

As sick as I was, I had been diagnosed quickly and treated immediately. That alone gave me a kind of privilege other kids didn't have.

I will never forget Cindy. She taught me about life, and she taught me about death. She was the first friend my own age I lost to cancer. I'll do everything I can to help raise awareness about childhood cancer until no one has to feel the pain I have felt. Not to mention that innocent lives are taken, and everyone who loves them is left behind to pick up the pieces.

Losing Cindy was a heartbreak that stayed with me deeply, but I soon learned that grief doesn't come alone. Just a month later, life dealt another heart-breaking blow. There had been this strong, beautiful young woman from my town, about my age, who had a similar diagnosis to me. Casey. I never had the honor of becoming real, in-person friends with her. We were only Facebook friends, where I followed her story. She lived life and was such an inspiring person already at her young age.

A huge day was coming for me. March 10, 2010. Since November 2007, it was a day I had looked forward to, dreamed about, doubted it would ever come, and counted down the days until. That was the day my treatment would officially be over. I would take my last chemo dose (hopefully forever) and move into follow-up care in place of active treatment.

All in all, my final dose was anticlimactic. There was a fraction of a pill (because a whole pill was overdosing me, which we learned quite late in my treatment) I was taking daily at that point, 6-MP (Mercaptopurine). It couldn't be taken within two hours of dairy or citrus, as those would interact with the active ingredient molecules and make it ineffective. That was a bummer, because I liked to take my pills with either Sunny D or milk since those overpowered the taste of the pills and helped everything slide down quickly. A different medicine was 13 tiny, nasty-tasting pills that dissolved immediately on my tongue, so I wanted them to go down as easily as possible.

Because of this, 6-MP was taken at night originally, after I had finished eating. I eventually moved it to the morning (slowly over time to not throw off taking it roughly 24 hours apart), as there are several times throughout the day I go without eating for four hours (two hours before and after), but the morning was much easier to take it on an empty stomach and not eat until lunch … since I did that most days anyway. Not eating two hours before bed was a little harder.

I woke up early in the morning, alone in my dorm room, swallowed the final dose, and was done. No fanfare. It didn't feel any different. I likely texted my family that I had just completed treatment because we recently had added texting to our phone plan (yes, that used to be a separate charge). But that was it.

The day carried on as normal. I got to live my life. It was the start of what I had been waiting for for almost two and a half years. I soon randomly started thinking about Casey. I was wondering what she was up to and was going to reach out to her to see if we could connect in person. Then I had one of those feelings in the pit of my stomach I didn't like.

When I went online, there were the words I was afraid of. Casey's obituary. She had passed away on March 10th. When I was celebrating (no matter how anticlimactic, it was still monumental) my end of treatment, she was at the end of her life. It didn't make sense. It wasn't fair. Any progress I had made since the month before when Cindy passed was immediately gone, and I sat at my desk, at my computer, and cried until I couldn't see clearly. Chest heaving, tears streaming down my face, and alone. Trying to make heads or tails of anything was futile.

Each loss reminded me of just how fragile life is, and how close I had come to facing the same fate. When my parents picked me up from school, I told them Casey had passed. I can only imagine what they were thinking. That that could have just as easily been me. And it will never make sense why it wasn't, but I've learned to stop asking why (most of the time). I'm embracing "doing good" as much as I can. Life and death are so randomly balanced. I had to live.

Despite the hospital's efforts to shield us from the harshest realities, grief was never far away—it lingered just beneath the surface, waiting to reveal itself in moments both quiet and devastating. You would see signs that the worst was happening. It might be the wail of a parent who just held their child for the last time shattering the silence of the hallway. Or the puffy red eyes on a tired parent's face that told you they were trying to keep it together in front of their kid, but were breaking on the inside and crying in private. Or the regulars you would see in the clinic or around the inpatient floor … until you didn't.

My heart goes out to every single person who has been touched by cancer. Especially every family that has imploded, forever changed by someone being ripped away from them. No child should die of cancer. No sibling should grow up without their brother or sister. No parent should have to bury their child. That is just unacceptable.

When I was at my sickest, I was scared of dying. I think most people are, at least to some extent. My biggest worry was what would happen to my family if I didn't make it. I'm so thankful they never had to face that.

Even something as small as worrying about the future of my toy bunny, Thumper, felt real. We joked about whether he would be buried with me or not. My family loves Thumper like he's one of us (we're a little weird, but if you ever met him, you'd see he has his own personality). Of course, I wouldn't let them lose two kids at once.

Looking back, these moments taught me so much about life, love, and loss. They showed me the fragility of our existence and the strength it takes to keep going.

But they also marked the beginning of something else— a complex feeling that would follow me long after treatment ended (that I've already mentioned a few times). Survivor's guilt.

That experience deserves its own story. So, in the next chapter—a bonus chapter—I'll share more about that complicated, often misunderstood, emotion.

For now, I'm grateful to be here, to be able to tell this story, and to keep honoring the memories of those who were lost along the way.

Chapter 7.5
Bonus Chapter: Survivor's Guilt

If you have ever experienced survivor's guilt, this is a special chapter just for you. If you haven't, feel free to skip ahead to the next chapter.

I'm not a trained psychologist—this chapter comes solely from my own experience. But if you think you need professional help, please reach out. Your medical team, social workers, or counselors can be a great place to start. Or even the internet, which has many resources at your fingertips. There may be support groups nearby, or one-on-one counseling that could be recommended.

Or maybe you're in a position where you can work through it with your close circle or even on your own. The caution with this is to know when you're in over your head. Remember that you are never alone. Many deal with survivor's guilt for various reasons, and there are people who care and want to help.

It's okay to talk about how you feel.

It's okay to cry or get angry.

It's okay to *feel*.

Everyone will die eventually. That doesn't mean each loss doesn't (or *shouldn't*) hurt. Some people are taken far too soon, which may bother us the most.

Survivor's guilt is because someone has died from a similar experience that you have survived, and you feel bad for doing so (as if you could have traded places with the other who did not make it). I can almost guarantee that your survival is in no way directly correlated with the death of someone else. Unless you murdered them … in which case you're likely not experiencing survivor's guilt, but your conscience …

Most deaths are not because only one person in the scenario can live (you're not Harry Potter or Voldemort).

Therefore, blaming yourself for living while another (or others) does not, will not do any good. It certainly will not bring anyone back.

This can lead you down dark rabbit holes that you can get lost in. If you ever have thoughts of hurting yourself, please reach out *immediately*—you don't have to face this alone. There are many services ready to help you, no matter where you live. Many can be found listed by country on www.suicide.org.

Try not to lose sight of the most important thing. You are here today. You are alive.

Your being here did not make it so someone else couldn't be. You didn't fill a seat on this Earth that booted someone else off it. There are likely reasons we will never understand for *"why?" "Why am I still here?" "Why isn't so-and-so here?" "Why did they die instead of me?"*

You will not get answers in this lifetime to these questions, so dwelling on them will not help anyone.

What personally helped me to stop focusing on *"why me?"* was when I decided to dedicate myself to being the best person I could be. This happened when my Make-A-Wish was granted. For me, volunteering and giving back to organizations such as Make-A-Wish has helped me to feel as if my life has a purpose. Again, this in no way means that anyone who lost or loses their battle did/does not have a purpose. I simply try to look at it as I (for whatever reason) was blessed with a second chance at life and have to utilize it to be my best self. My journey isn't over yet, and I have to make that worthwhile.

Your journey is also not over.

Your story does not end here.

What you do with it next is up to you.

If you know someone who is experiencing survivor's guilt, be there for them.

Listen.

Allow them time to grieve for the person or people they have lost.

You may not understand what they are experiencing. That's okay. If they trust you enough to let you in on what is going on (to any extent), that is probably a good thing.

Perhaps you're someone they feel comfortable confiding in. Possibly they're reaching out for help (either to work through their emotions independently or beginning to seek outside assistance).

Don't push them away. They are likely in quite a vulnerable state.

Maybe they aren't fully ready to talk about everything they are feeling. Don't force them or they might shut down entirely.

I also would not recommend invalidating their feelings or telling them to "snap out of it."

Survivor's guilt is a serious and potentially crippling state.

Instead, nurture them in whatever way is normal for your relationship. Remind them how important they are to your life and how happy you are to have them here.

An important thing is to recognize when you should encourage this person to get professional help (if it comes to this point). Also, do not be afraid to seek out some yourself (even if you just need assistance getting your loved one the help they need).

If you haven't experienced survivor's guilt (and I know I said you could skip this chapter), I hope you never have to.

If you are dealing with survivor's guilt, may you find what works for you, and make the most out of your time on this planet.

I'm very glad you're here.

Chapter 8
Second Chances

We often don't fully appreciate what we have until it's gone. And usually, by that point, it's too late—it's lost forever.

But sometimes, we're given second chances. Those rare moments when we get back something we thought was gone for good. When that happens, we shouldn't make the same mistake twice. Instead, we should hold on, always remembering how fortunate we are to have that blessing in our lives—because we know how quickly it could be taken away.

These unexpected gifts of grace have taught me to never take even the smallest blessings for granted. Throughout my journey, there were a few moments where I was given another shot at something I thought was lost forever.

The biggest? Life itself.

No one is promised tomorrow—not even the healthiest among us. But the moment it truly clicked for me just how fragile life was happened the day my lumbar puncture sedation went wrong—and I almost didn't wake up. Just like that, it could have all been over.

After that, I started living each day differently. I treated every moment like it was not only my last but my very first. I embraced life with a childlike wonder that still stays with me. Knowing that life could end at any time, I do my best to appreciate every second. I seize every opportunity and chase after what brings me joy while I still can.

I'm aware that there might come a day when I'm not as well as I am now—I've already faced that reality. So if something exciting comes my way, I go for it. Take London, for example. In the decade after my Make-A-Wish was granted, I returned roughly every other year. Whenever I'd tell people I was going again, they'd say, "Again?" *Absolutely!* As long as I'm fortunate enough to have the means and the desire, I will keep going. London is a place where I feel at home—a place that makes me happy. Who wouldn't want that feeling?

But appreciating life isn't just about the big adventures. It's also about celebrating the small victories—like something as simple as climbing stairs.

There was quite a long stretch of time during my treatment and recovery when I simply couldn't walk up or down stairs. I don't remember exactly when I first managed to do it again, but I am endlessly grateful that I can now. That ability—something so basic and often taken for granted— became a meaningful milestone in my journey. Whenever possible, I choose to take the stairs rather than the elevator. It's a small way to celebrate the strength and progress I've regained, even if it's only two floors.

I teach on the third floor of my school, which actually means climbing about four flights of stairs because of how the building was designed—essentially two flights between each floor. I make it a point to walk those stairs every time I need to go up or down, unless there's some truly exceptional circumstance. It might seem insignificant to most people, but to me, those flights of stairs represent something much bigger: reclaiming a part of my independence and normal life. Yet, despite my commitment to taking the stairs, I often get asked, "Why don't you take the elevator?" or people assume that I do. It's just two floors, and as long as I'm physically able, I will keep choosing the stairs. It feels like a quiet victory.

Running, on the other hand, has never been something I naturally did or enjoyed. If you've ever met me—before, during, or after cancer—the word "runner" probably wouldn't come to mind. Unless, of course, you were trying to think of what I'm definitely not. I don't run. I wasn't built for it, never have been, and never really liked it. But I was capable of it—sort of. Usually only when it was a matter of life or death. For instance, if I was being chased by a wasp (which terrifies me to this day) or if the last pieces of fried chicken were up for grabs at a buffet, those were the rare moments when you'd see me "run," or at least jog in desperation.

Back in the day, I could "run" a mile in about twelve minutes—though that time is certainly up for debate and probably closer to a brisk walk than anything else. Now, I'd guess it would take me closer to fifteen minutes to cover the same distance jogging. Honestly, I might be able to powerwalk a mile faster than I could run it these days. If that's even possible.

When my body finally told me that running was no longer an option, that hit me hard. It was frustrating, disheartening, and just plain unfair. Then came the medical reality check: after my treatment, it would take roughly a year for the chemotherapy toxins to fully clear my system. Side effects caused by the medication—especially the ones affecting nerve and muscle function, like my inability to run—could improve during that time. But after the year was up, any lingering side effects were likely permanent. That was a tough pill to swallow.

And there was still the issue of "foot drop" and the jelly-like uncertainty that made my legs feel like they might give out without warning. My brain wanted to move faster than my legs were capable of, and that disconnect often caused me to stumble or fall—even during my usual quick-paced walks. It was concerning, especially because I had to remind myself constantly that I couldn't run. If I forgot, and something urgent happened—like a wasp chase—my legs might fail me, and I'd faceplant.

I realized I had a window of opportunity, a critical year to push my body as much as possible to regain strength and reverse whatever damage I could. So I started walking around the indoor track at my university's athletic center. It wasn't as easy as it sounds, but I needed to rebuild my confidence in my legs. Then one day, my legs suddenly felt stronger. They didn't tremble as much. They seemed ready. Ready to try jogging again.

With all that in mind, I cautiously tried a few strides. My shins burned from muscles unused to the exertion, but I didn't fall. I kept going. Step by step, I pushed myself to complete a full lap around the small track. When I finished, I leaned over, gasping for breath, trying to calm my pounding heart.

I was ecstatic.

To anyone watching, it might have been the slowest, saddest lap ever, but to me, it was a triumph. For the first time in years, I had jogged again—a simple thing I never imagined I'd do after everything I'd been through.

Did this moment turn me into a runner or marathon hopeful? Absolutely not. But it was a victory nonetheless. I'm incredibly grateful that I can "run" when I want or need to. It's a reminder of how far I've come, and how much strength I can still find inside me.

Physical recovery wasn't just about jogging laps. Regaining hand strength was another hard-fought battle, and every small victory—whether it was climbing stairs, holding a pencil firmly, or opening a jar—became a precious reminder that my body was healing and that second chances really were possible.

My hands were incredibly weak and sore during treatment, which made even the simplest tasks frustrating. My handwriting became messy and illegible, and there were times when I could barely use my hands at all. But as the medicines gradually worked their way out of my system, things improved dramatically. While I still have some lingering cramps and occasional spasms that can be strong enough to cause me to drop things unexpectedly, it's a million times better than it used to be. My handwriting, for example, is almost as good as it was before treatment. Sure, I can't write for hours on end without my hands cramping up, and it takes more effort to make my writing look neat, but I can do it—and that feels like a huge win. The biggest minor inconvenience I can't really complain about is that I still usually can't open jars or bottles by myself—like opening a simple water bottle is a struggle. But hey, isn't that what my husband is for? I joke, but it's honestly just one of those little things I've had to accept. Overall, my hand function has come so far compared to what it could have been, and I'm grateful for that every day.

While my hands improved significantly, the nerve damage didn't stop there. Another challenge was the injury to a nerve in my right thigh, which brought a whole different set of struggles. At first, I was told that part of the nerve was so badly injured that it would never heal. It was a brutal thing to hear and even harder to accept. The sensation in that part of my leg went through stages. Initially, I couldn't feel anything—complete numbness. Then came the "asleep" feeling, with sharp pins and needles that sometimes made even light clothing feel unbearable. The numbness and prickly tingling sensations would alternate, leaving me in a constant state of discomfort and uncertainty.

Eventually, that numbness evolved into a cold, dead feeling—like my leg tissue was there, but lifeless. The awful pins and needles would still come and go, like my body was desperately trying to "wake up" the leg after its long slumber. Just when I started resigning myself to the idea that this would be permanent, something miraculous began to happen. In the rotation of sensations, I started having moments where I could feel my leg without the sharp pain. These moments would come and go, mingling with numbness and the occasional pins and needles, but those glimpses of normal sensation felt incredible.

Now, as I'm writing this, I'd say my right leg feels about 80% normal compared to my left—especially during those "good moments" when the sensation is almost like it was before the nerve injury. I still get the numbness and pins and needles, but those stretches of semi-normal feeling are wonderful—and I don't take them for granted, especially after hearing the initial prognosis that my leg would never improve. It's one of those second chances I'm endlessly thankful for.

Just as my nerves were slowly getting better, I was faced with another physical challenge that felt as daunting: the limited use of my shoulders.

After my Make-A-Wish was granted, I kept improving—sometimes in ways doctors said were impossible. During my wish trip, and honestly within the very first day, I decided I was going to study abroad the following summer. I didn't tell my family right away because I knew they might try to talk me out of it, especially since it meant spending most of my life savings. I wanted to be absolutely sure before I officially applied to the program.

The idea of going to another country alone was terrifying—not just because it was a foreign place, but because I wasn't even sure if I was physically capable of doing it.

London, thankfully, is much more handicap accessible than many American cities. But it's no step-free paradise. (Back then, stairs were still a slow, painstaking process for me.) This was on top of very limited use of my shoulders because of the avascular necrosis (AVN), which caused constant pain. I couldn't lift my arms over my head—not something you think about until you realize just how often that motion is needed, especially if you're as short as I am. And to add to the challenge, one of my doctors warned me not to lift too much weight to avoid putting extra strain on my already overworked heart. So, lugging around a heavy suitcase full of books and chocolate by the end of my trip? *Don't ask* ... Not ideal.

Put all of that together and you had a petite young woman who couldn't run from danger, climbed stairs slowly and carefully, couldn't lift her arms high, and probably couldn't carry her own suitcases for very long. Honestly, there was every reason to be nervous about me traveling alone.

But those nine months between my Make-A-Wish and studying abroad were all about preparation. I pushed myself, doing what I could to get stronger—cardio workouts and strength training within my limits. Slowly but surely, my shoulders started to improve.

When it came time to get on the plane, I did it by myself. I carried my heavy carry-on bag—the one with my eight-pound laptop inside for the class I was taking—and, for the first time in what felt like forever, I lifted it over my head to put it into the overhead compartment. For someone who's only five feet tall, that's quite the stretch. *Literally.* But I did it. That moment was huge for me. It was proof I was going to be okay. I had done something I never thought I would again—lifted a heavy object over my head and gotten it safely into a space much higher than me. When we landed, I managed to get the bag down on my own, too. It hurt a little, mainly because gravity seemed to have more control over my suitcase than I did, but I still did it. Up and down, on my own.

That might sound trivial or like no big deal if you're someone who's never lost that ability. But for me, it was monumental. It was a reminder of how much I'd regained and how much I still had to appreciate. From that day on, I promised myself never to take lifting my arms pain-free over my head for granted again—because there was a time when that simple movement felt impossible.

Alongside all the physical challenges, the hospital surprisingly became a place where my creativity could flourish—a crucial part of my healing process. The eighth floor of Connecticut Children's Medical Center wasn't just a ward; it became more of a second home than anywhere else I had been. I looked forward to the weekly activities they offered because they gave me a break from thinking about being sick. Of course, you had to be feeling well enough to enjoy them, but when I was, there was always something interesting going on. Some activities happened in community spaces, but others came right to your hospital room, which was especially comforting when your family couldn't be there because they were at work or school. The people who organized and led these events—mostly volunteers, I believe—were so kind and genuinely wonderful.

Two activities I really got into were photography and scrapbooking. The photography volunteer had a beautiful camera you got to use during the session, and at the end, they would print the pictures you took. Even though I was stuck within the four walls of the hospital, I found endless inspiration to capture through the lens. This sparked a real interest in photography for me, and shortly after, I got my own fancy camera. (Now, of course, cell phones have incredible cameras built right in, making photography so much more accessible.) Scrapbooking was another activity that grabbed my attention and inspired a hobby that has stuck with me ever since—I even made one scrapbook filled with all the photos I took during my hospital stay.

There were other fun and creative activities, too. I remember using GarageBand to make music—which was exciting since I had taken a music production class the year before and enjoyed working with the program. Another craft was making pins; I made one that said "cancer sucks" with a little lollipop drawn on it—a perfect *taste* of my sense of humor—and I proudly wore it on my hat. Other volunteers encouraged me to try painting and drawing. I wasn't amazing at those, but I gave it my best shot (still think I stink at it, honestly). One volunteer even inspired me to explore writing, which eventually led to *Thumper's Adventures*, as well as a few other children's cancer book ideas I haven't fully pursued yet. Occasionally, first-run movies would come directly from the distributors on VHS (yup, I'm that old) so we could watch them since getting to a cinema wasn't an option.

The hospital team did everything they could to keep us happy and distracted. There was a cozy playroom with an air hockey table, a little oasis for kids who could get out of their rooms. Remember, this was before smartphones and tablets were everywhere, so the entertainment options were different. TVs were in every room, and there were some fancier electronics—like game systems or laptops—you could borrow for a while. I sometimes used a laptop to check in on Facebook and update a site called CaringBridge, which was specifically designed to keep family and friends posted on your medical journey. It was like a digital journal where visitors could leave messages of support. Looking back, given how technology was still pretty clunky at the time and how overwhelmed we were, it would have been nice to keep a more real-time record of everything. Many people wanted to know how we were doing, and having that ongoing communication would have been helpful—not just for others but also as a record for us. But honestly, we were just focused on surviving. We simply didn't have the energy or bandwidth to keep up with technology (plus, my family still isn't very tech savvy even now).

While these distractions helped, it was my passion for acting that truly became a lifeline during those difficult days. Acting has always been a big part of who I am, and throughout this journey, it grew even more important. It gave me a sense of purpose, a way to escape, and a connection to the life I wanted to live beyond the hospital walls.

About two weeks after my diagnosis, the school play I was originally—perhaps delusionally—convinced I would still be able to act in had its opening night. My family took me to see the performance, and my friends along with the Drama Club were incredibly thoughtful—they cleared out a section of the auditorium just for us so I could sit without being near anyone who might make me sicker. That was my first big outing since the diagnosis, and it was a lot to take in. We only made it through intermission before I was too fatigued to stay any longer and had to head home. Thankfully, the performance was filmed, and I was able to watch the rest of the show later on. I'm so grateful to everyone who helped make that experience possible and especially to the person who stepped in at the last minute to take over my role so the show could go on. Their kindness meant the world to me.

As the months passed, I found myself missing acting and the sense of purpose and joy it brought me. I had to practically beg my doctors to let me be involved in the spring musical, especially since I wasn't even physically at school anymore and was relying on homebound tutoring. But eventually, they understood how important it was for my mental health and gave me permission. I was allowed to join the chorus for one song in the spring production of *Annie*. It certainly wasn't a big role but just being part of a cast, rehearsing, and performing was amazing. It gave me something positive to focus on, a welcome distraction from everything else going on in my life. That small taste of normalcy was so necessary for me.

Being able to act again, even in a limited way, was a haven. It helped keep my spirits up when things felt bleak. I chose to focus on the positives because it helped my overall attitude and outlook on life.

Inspired by that, I developed a daily practice that has been essential for staying grounded through all the ups and downs of life.

For the past several years, I've kept a thankfulness journal. Every night before bed, I write down at least three things I'm grateful for. Some days that's easier than others, but I never skip it. Sometimes the things I jot down seem silly or small, but they all matter. On the roughest days, I find that even the absence of something negative—like a day without pain or discomfort—counts as a blessing. For instance, one time, a deer suddenly darted in front of my car, and although it was terrifying, I was grateful I didn't hit it. Even during one of the worst days of my life, when my dad suffered a massive heart attack, I focused on the fact that it was caught in time and that he was able to come home just a few days later. And that I had my brother to keep me sane through all the waiting. Those small sparks of hope and gratitude have helped me keep going.

No matter what life throws at me, I try to focus on the positives. It's a conscious choice every single day.

This mindset—of focusing on what I have rather than what I've lost—helps me recognize just how incredibly fortunate I am. Despite everything cancer took from me, I've been blessed with so many second chances. Cancer stole countless things from my life, but the ones I got back, I'll never take for granted again.

Chapter 9
Finding the Silver Lining

Does everything happen for a reason? I don't believe bad things necessarily happen on purpose, but I do believe that good can always come out of even the darkest moments.

Cancer brought with it an avalanche of challenges— pain, fear, and uncertainty. But alongside all that, it also opened unexpected doors to incredible people I might never have met otherwise. The most profound of those connections were with other survivors. From the moment of diagnosis until your last breath, you're considered a survivor, part of a community bonded by shared fears, hopes, and resilience. Because of my journey, I was honored to grow close to a few remarkable people I otherwise might never have known. Though that closeness came with its own heartbreaks, I wouldn't trade those experiences.

Cancer provides a connection that crosses all ages and backgrounds. Even if it's a different form or stage, when I meet someone who's fighting this disease, there's an unspoken kinship. We relate on a deep level. Our challenges might be unique, but we've all grappled with similar thoughts and fears.

That kinship became utterly personal midway through my treatment, when one of my cousins was diagnosed with a brain tumor. I'll never forget that she asked to see me. Of everyone she could have asked for, she wanted me. At first, I didn't understand why—and then I did. We were both facing cancer. *Duh.*

I walked into her dark hospital room, saw her lying there uncertain of what the next day would bring, and it clicked just how similar we were. I don't remember exactly what we said during that visit, but in that half hour, we grew closer than we had ever been. She's faced obstacles since, but it's been over a decade now (*knock on wood*).

About a year after I finished treatment, a family friend was diagnosed with Stage 4 stomach cancer. Once again, that shared experience of cancer brought us closer.

When he first told us, you'd never have guessed he was already in the middle of a life-or-death battle. Every time I saw him, he'd fist bump me and ask how I was doing. At that point, I was fine. He was so optimistic he'd beat his cancer, and he told me I was inspiring him to keep fighting.

For some reason, that stung.

Maybe it was guilt. Or the unfairness of it all. Or the ache of knowing optimism doesn't always change outcomes. In moments like that, I felt like an imposter. Though I'd come close to losing my fight, fortune had been on my side. I had a high survival rate, never relapsed (*knock on wood*), didn't need a bone marrow transplant (*knock on wood*), and only had chemotherapy without radiation.

Maybe it was the cynic in me staring down the single-digit chance of survival he faced and preparing for the worst. Of course, I never said that out loud and prayed I was wrong. I hoped he'd be one to beat the odds.

Sadly, that wasn't meant to be. He passed away a few months later.

Despite heartbreaks, I've continued to meet other survivors—some newly diagnosed, others far along in recovery. It's kind of amazing how quickly you can form a bond with someone who's faced cancer. Not everyone wants to talk about their medical history, and sharing that experience doesn't automatically make you best friends. But I've had many touching, therapeutic conversations with those willing to open up.

I'm grateful for every person cancer brought into my life—and I carry those it took from me even closer in my heart.

Through it all, the people who stood by me every step of the way—through every high, low, and everything in between—was my family.

I'm eternally grateful to have such a loving, tight-knit group in my corner. We're always there for each other, spending quality time together. We do our fair share of yelling and screaming too, but that's part of what keeps us close. We don't bottle things up. We tell each other straight out when something's wrong so we can work through it and move on. It's not always quiet, but it works—and it has kept us strong.

That strength was tested from the moment I was diagnosed.

Doctors warned us many families fall apart under the pressure of childhood cancer—that parents often split, overwhelmed by stress. That was *exactly* what I needed to hear at the time. As if fighting for my life wasn't enough, I might also be the reason our family fell apart.

Thankfully, the opposite happened. If anything, we pulled even closer—though that meant spending a lot of time in my cold, cave-like hospital room. (I was always too hot and sensitive to light, so the room was kept dim and chilly.)

One person who was always there was my brother, D.J. We've always been close, but when I got sick, our bond only grew stronger. Whether I wanted to play Yahtzee for the millionth time in the middle of the night, needed help applying lotion to my dry feet (yes, he did that ... with gloves, but he did it!), or just wanted company on evenings when our parents couldn't stay over, he was there. He even visited when he was on a break from law school work nearby in Hartford.

He was also there to have fun when I was up for it. After I got out of the hospital, he started taking me to musicals at The Bushnell. We saw a few amazing shows (and one ... *interesting* ... rendition). Those nights out were pure delight and will always be special to me. When I was in college, I won tickets to see *The Lion King*, and it was my turn to take my brother to a show. He even joined me for some teen group activities like indoor mini golf. And once, we attended a cancer summit in New York City together.

Our adventures will always hold a special place in my heart.

When I needed "liquid" medicine administered at home—whether through a shot or my port—D.J. was always on top of it. My dad took care of the medicines that could be given "hands-off," while D.J. took charge of the injections. No matter what I needed—distraction, care, or simply someone to sit with me—he showed up. Gloves and all.

Of course, none of this would have been possible without my parents, who were always there in the background—and often the foreground—keeping everything running. They supported each other (and me) by tag-teaming my care alongside everything else that had to happen to keep life moving forward. My dad organized and prepared the thousands of pills I had to take at all hours. He worked tirelessly to make sure my health insurance never lapsed, so I could continue receiving the remarkable care I needed to survive. My mom worked a few days a week as a preschool teacher but was with me whenever she wasn't working, staying over most nights.

Not everyone has that kind of support, and I will never stop being grateful that I did. They didn't just help me survive—they helped me live through it.

While my family was the foundation that held me up during treatment, I was also lifted by the strength of my community. As word of my diagnosis spread, friends, neighbors, and even strangers showed up in ways I never expected.

One of the most memorable moments came during my town's first Relay for Life, just a few months after I began treatment. My friends formed a team to support me—Team Dexter, named after my first IV pole—and everyone got involved. It was an incredible night at the high school track, raising money for cancer research. Luminaries lined the path to honor survivors and remember those lost to the disease. The goal was to "outwalk cancer," with someone from each team walking the entire event.

There was a movie shown on the lawn, people camping out, and various other activities.

As much as I wanted to stay through the night, fatigue and cold eventually got the better of me. I was still too sick for sleeping outdoors to be safe—or comfortable—so I had to head home.

My dad walked. The. Whole. Time.

I never asked him why, but I imagine he felt that was the one thing he could control. He didn't have a say in whether I got cancer or not, nor in whether I lived or died. But maybe if he could walk the whole event, I would be able to make it, too. Maybe he really could outwalk cancer. *My* cancer.

Even years later, people in town still talk about that first Relay. It was beautiful to see everyone come together. A few people even still remember how my dad walked the whole time.

The following year, the event moved to a larger venue because it had outgrown the high school. It was miraculous to witness and be part of. As I grew stronger and healthier each year, I became more involved in the planning committee. I felt driven to help other survivors and cancer research—and this was a good place to start. My brother joined, too, and we worked on it together for a few years.

There was a whole aspect of the event dedicated to survivors, celebrating those going through treatment as well as those who had completed it. I felt deeply connected to that part and helped organize survivor events, even giving a few speeches. It was great to connect with people from town or nearby who participated and were also survivors. Some I had known, others I met through the Relay.

In the beginning, everyone was further out from treatment than I was, as I was still actively undergoing treatment in those first few years. Once, just twenty-four hours after my port was removed, I participated. I thought it was amazing to be up and moving, doing something to help other survivors so soon after surgery—especially compared to how hard the port placement surgery had been. As the years went on, others recently diagnosed began their journeys, while I had entered post-treatment life.

The Relays were a blast, and I hold those memories dear. Eventually, my town stopped hosting them. I could have joined another town's event, but it didn't feel the same. This was the community that had walked with me through it all—our Relay.

Around that time, my attention shifted toward another cause that had become close to my heart: Make-A-Wish.

During my involvement in the Relay, I was waiting for my own wish to be granted. When my wish finally came true, I felt a strong pull to give back to Make-A-Wish. It was the right time—especially since the Relay had moved on to other communities. (Not that you can't support multiple charities at once—I just tend to go "all in" when I commit to something.)

I also feel a strong drive to support more focused research for childhood cancer. When I was first diagnosed, I naively assumed all cancers received equal funding and research opportunities. But childhood cancer is grossly underfunded. Yes, some other cancers face similar challenges, but childhood cancer affects a crucial part of the population—kids. As my journey continued, I learned just how underserved this area is, and I wanted to help change that. That's why a portion of this book's proceeds goes toward fighting childhood cancer. I still support the Relay for Life organization and might get involved again someday, but right now, I dedicate much of my energy and time to other causes—and I don't regret any of those decisions.

Alongside charity work, I found another outlet for reflection and expression—writing.

I first discovered *CURE* magazine while waiting at the clinic. It's a free publication for cancer patients and caregivers, full of research updates, personal stories, and advice. One article, about the role of the arts during treatment, moved me enough to write a letter to the editor.

To my surprise, they published part of my letter. It felt surreal—thousands of readers, and somehow my words made it in. A few years later, they published another letter from me, and even a short essay on their website. I wasn't playing the "cancer card"—just sharing my truth, like so many others do. It's pretty cool to see your words in print. I suppose that's part of why I enjoy writing books.

That wasn't my only unexpected brush with publishing—or broadcasting, for that matter.

While recovering at home, I found comfort in something familiar: an educational children's TV show. *Yes ... I sometimes watch children's shows.* This one is surprisingly thoughtful, even for adults. One day, they announced a contest for kids to create a new character. I was definitely too old, but I emailed them anyway, pitching a character with cancer.

I figured it could help kids understand cancer better—what it means, how it's not contagious, and that the person going through it is still the same on the inside. They emailed back to say it was a great idea—and encouraged me to enter the contest. I guess they missed the part where I admitted I was over the age limit.

About a year later, they released a two-part episode featuring a character diagnosed with cancer. They handled it beautifully—just how I hoped. The episodes covered emotional and physical changes, explained fear and uncertainty, and emphasized that the person going through it is still them.

It might've just been a coincidence, but I like to believe I had a small part in that moment.

That wasn't the only time I suggested something a TV show may or may not have drawn from, which is pretty cool.

But I did get to contribute in a more official and scientific setting. Besides the clinical study I participated in during treatment, I had the chance to join another research program afterward. This one focused on late-term effects on the heart, since one of the chemotherapy drugs is known to cause issues down the line. It involved exercise, bloodwork, physical fitness tests, and lab work before, during, and after the study.

I signed up not knowing if I'd be able to complete it—because, honestly, I don't exactly do high strenuous exercise. The study required exercising several times a week over a few months.

I went in with low expectations for myself but was determined to push through. I wanted to help in any way I could so something good might come from my experience. The more we learn, the better treatment and survivorship will be for future cancer patients.

The study turned out great for me—I made it through. The gym membership they provided encouraged me to exercise, and the regular fitness tests kept me accountable. Along the way, I made an incredible friend and found a few classes I truly enjoyed—one I continued even after the membership ended, joining virtually during the pandemic lockdown. I haven't kept up as much as I'd like, but I know I can if I find the willpower again. That means something.

Throughout all my experiences, I gained a deeper appreciation for the people who make pediatric hospitals feel like more than just medical buildings.

It takes a special kind of person to work in a children's hospital, especially with hematology and oncology patients. Kids are our future; they're just at the dawn of life. To see them suffering—and some not surviving—takes a truly remarkable person to do that work. I have immense respect for everyone who chooses that path.

There were moments I considered switching from my lifelong dream of becoming a teacher to maybe becoming a pediatric oncology nurse. But then I thought about all that would entail. I get attached to inanimate objects (like my beloved Thumper) and struggle to say goodbye even for short times to the people I love. I'm not built to face the heartbreaking cycle of children losing their medical battles. No one should have to endure that, as no child should have to die from a medical condition. It's idealistic, but it's a vision I'll do everything I can to help make real.

Everyone my family met along the way was fantastic. My nurses felt like family. It was always a good day if my regular in the clinic was there. Or my inpatient stays were always that much easier when I'd see certain names on the whiteboards. But it was impossible to have favorites when everyone who cared for me in the clinic or MS8 was so incredible.

I loved my primary oncologist, but they all took turns checking in, each bringing something unique. One once brought a guitar and played a holiday song for my mom and me while I was inpatient. Another, a pediatric oncologist who had served in the Air Force and flown planes, eventually became my doctor when mine moved away. How cool is that? A hero in two jobs.

And then there were the people who supported us emotionally—especially our social worker. She had the softest heart and the fiercest dedication.

Another major part of my support system was the teen group, led by Christine (aka "Scary Doll Lady") and Sarah. Somehow, they transformed a cancer support group into something that was actually fun. It felt odd at first, since I was pretty much the only girl who attended and seemed to be the only one still in treatment. But that changed over time.

I remember one of the first events was around Christmas. There was a boy who had just finished treatment for the same cancer I had just started. Everyone was celebrating that he was done. I wanted so badly to be happy for him (and part of me was), but I'm ashamed to admit I was jealous. That's not something I feel often—I'm usually good about being happy for others without wanting what they have. But this hit differently. It wasn't just that he was done and I was only beginning treatment. I didn't know *if* I would make it to the end. If I did, it would be two and a half years away—which felt like forever. But the *"would I make it?"* part was the worst.

A few months into treatment, there was a group meeting while I was in the hospital. Most meetings took place in the evening so kids living outpatient lives could attend. At this one, there was a girl with a beautiful short haircut. Again, I felt that green-eyed monster of envy—I had some ugly feelings inside I'm not proud of—that this time was entirely misplaced. Her hair was gorgeous, and I had recently lost most of mine. I assumed she was near the end of her treatment and getting her life back together.

But I was wrong.

I soon learned she had just been diagnosed on Christmas Eve. While I had just gotten home and was able to enjoy some normal aspects of a "Merry Christmas," her family was in the hospital with their lives falling apart. She was also a twin. Natalie became a good friend, as we had similar journeys and could talk about experiences no one else really understood.

With the teen group, we had enjoyable outings—like cliff jumping—and a Christmas party where all the families got together. Yes, my cancer support group took us cliff jumping. It was at an extreme water park with activities like zip lining into the water, sliding from high drops, bouncing off the "blob," or jumping from cliffs into the water. *Hey, we survived cancer, so why not jump off a cliff because everyone else was doing it?* It was liberating (and obviously safe—otherwise, they wouldn't encourage customers to jump). It was important we did this as a group, but one at a time, since all at once would be *too* dangerous. We had all faced (or were still facing) our battles, but this was a moment where we could take control, run to the cliff's edge, and jump.

In that moment when I leapt—to what could have been my death (but I tend to trust people maybe too much)—for one brief moment, it felt as if I could fly. Until dependable gravity plummeted me deep into the water. It felt like I could do anything. It was wonderful. I don't think I'll be finding other cliffs to jump from any time soon, but I'm slightly interested in parachuting from an airplane (one meant for that, not because it's your only exit).

That exhilarating sense of freedom and control was something I rarely felt during treatment. But there were other moments—more grounded yet just as joyful—that helped me find normalcy and connection. At the annual Christmas party, we'd build gingerbread houses. I don't remember if it started as a competition, or if D.J. and I made it into one. We're both very "things have to be as perfect and organized as possible" people, so building gingerbread houses turned into an art form. Getting the walls (or one year, a train) to stay together was the hardest part. Some other groups started decorating before their houses were stable, and they'd collapse. Who really cares, right? They were having fun. *D.J. and I cared.* At least about our project. We got the walls and roof stable, and only then did the color-coded, well-thought-out decorating begin. Our house (or train) would usually look like a well-organized rainbow exploded on it by the end.

While gingerbread house building fed my need for precision and creativity, the hospital also gave us chances to enjoy team spirit and cheer together. About once a year, we'd go to a Wolf Pack game (professional hockey). Someone generous donated a box for the hospital, and we got to watch from the private box with a buffet of food. I'm not going to lie—that was an awesome experience (and I'm not a typical sports fan).

Among all the outings, one stands out as particularly memorable—not for grandeur, but for the simple joy and camaraderie it brought. It was right on my birthday (April 1st) at a restaurant and arcade: Chuck E. Cheese. We did this *for* my birthday. We basically had unlimited tokens to play games, which was so much fun. I'd only been there before with limited tokens (which I always appreciated), so having free rein was awesome.

Amid the fun and distractions, there were also moments that made me reflect deeply on my experiences—like when we were asked to imagine how a better clinic might look. Toward the end of my treatment, I remember one meeting where they asked what I would do if I was in charge of designing a new oncology clinic. At the time, I thought it was just a random exercise to help us reflect on our experiences. I didn't realize we were essentially a focus group. I would have given very different answers had I known a new clinic was actually in the works. I remember they asked what I would name the new clinic, and without a better idea, I said "Pink Fluffy Star"—because I was special. The hospital did build a new clinic (5A), which opened a little while later.

I have such wonderful memories of those gatherings. In the midst of uncertainty and scary moments, that group felt like a refuge. Everyone deserves a place where they feel they belong—a place where people truly understand and accept them for who they are. For me, teen group was exactly that. I hope supports like it still exist, not just at CCMC, but in every hospital.

Once treatment was behind me and I finished college, a sense of gratitude fueled a sense of purpose for me. The urge to give back. I knew I had to become the best version of myself and not waste this second chance at life I was given. As long as I'm here, I want to make the world a brighter, better place.

I became a teacher, something I had always dreamed of. I'd like to think that through teaching, I'm doing some good for future generations. Each time a student tells me they enjoy our class or comes back years later (yes … I'm already old) to say how it inspired them, it means the world to me. I've always believed that children are our future. The more energy and care we invest in them—whether it's education, healthcare, food, or housing—the better all our futures will be.

Beyond the classroom, I continued to find other ways to give back: volunteering. I pay forward the incredible gift I once received by volunteering with Make-A-Wish. Considering they gave me (quite literally) the world and played a crucial part during my treatment, helping other children is the least I can do.

Through volunteering, I've met extraordinary people and helped grant over forty wishes so far. I love meeting each wish kid and connecting with their families. The greatest joy comes when a wish is granted, and I see the same happiness light up their faces that I once experienced. That joy lasts far longer than a single day. Wishes create lifelong memories for the entire family.

But volunteering isn't always sunshine and butterflies. Children eligible for Make-A-Wish face critical illnesses, which carries a profound sadness. While we bring a spark of joy to families during incredibly difficult times, not every child gets better (though many do grow up and live long, healthy lives).

Every wish kid I've lost has cut deep. You grow to love the child and their family and root for them to beat every odd stacked against them. When a child passes away, it never gets easier. Families are forever changed. Siblings grow up without their best friend. Parents carry on without their child.

I've witnessed firsthand how the Make-A-Wish experience continues to bring comfort even after a wish child passes. Whether it's a tangible thing left behind—like a backyard sanctuary families can visit to feel close to their child—or the treasured memories of that magical time, I've never seen a family who didn't look back fondly on their wish. That's part of the true magic of Make-A-Wish.

Every day, I'm reminded how my story could have ended differently. On my way to and from work, I pass through an intersection where two wish families lived—families who have had to go on without their children. Both kids were close to my age and had similar diagnoses, both from my hometown. Since I started volunteering, I've taken on as many of my hometown wish kids as I can because I feel such a special connection.

The similarities are too many to ignore. Either one could have been me. Either family could have been mine.

My heart goes out to them every single day. They're never far from my thoughts. I'm so sorry their stories didn't have happier endings.

Most of my time volunteering with Make-A-Wish is filled with happy moments. I have the honor of helping kids figure out what their true wish is and seeing the process through until it's granted.

My wish kids have incredible, creative, and always special wishes. Trips to Disney World, Disneyland, Italy to meet family, New Zealand to visit *The Lord of the Rings* filming locations, London to meet favorite actors, Summer Slam, Atlantis, Hawaii, Universal …

Wishes for backyard makeovers to create safe, private spaces for hanging out with friends and family. Parties to celebrate life and family. Electronics like iPads or unique virtual reality systems. Shopping sprees—both local and destination.

The list keeps growing with every wish.

I've met the strongest kids and their wonderful families—people facing the unimaginable with such grace (way more than I ever had). They balance the weight of the world on their shoulders while juggling everyday life's other responsibilities. Each family holds a special place in my heart—I have many special places in my heart, after all. I treasure the time they share with me and thank them for welcoming me into their journey, even if only for a small part.

I could go on and on about these heroes, but their stories belong to them—not me.

I've also had the chance to volunteer alongside inspiring wish granters and Make-A-Wish employees. People who go above and beyond their job descriptions to make each wish as magical as possible—surpassing even the wildest imaginations. Some of these amazing folks are previous wish kids, like me. Others are wish parents, siblings, grandparents, aunts, uncles, cousins, friends … and then there are those remarkable souls with no direct connection to Make-A-Wish at all. They've never been touched by a wish but somehow felt called to help anyway. That's one of the most inspiring things to me.

For someone like me, who's been on the receiving end of a wish, it's easy to give back. But for someone with no personal connection to jump in? That's truly amazing.

The Make-A-Wish family is a wonderful collection of people from all walks of life, united by one mission: to grant the wish of every eligible child.

In addition to wish granting—where I work directly with families—I help out at events like the annual gala, one of our biggest fundraisers. Wish kids get to interact with sponsors, and I love reconnecting with families I've worked with before, as well as meeting new ones.

If there's ever anything else I can help with, my answer is "yes." Whether it's a two-hour round trip to the Make-A-Wish office for a trunk-or-treat event, attending a sunflower fundraiser in the summer, or literally anything else they need. If I can do it, I will.

When a wish involves local activities, wish granters often help on the day of the wish itself. I've escorted kids on shopping sprees, planning routes, communicating with stores so managers can do special things (which many do, going above and beyond), and carrying bags. It's a joy to see a child's eyes light up like they're in a candy store—sometimes literally, since candy stops are occasionally on the list—knowing they can have anything their heart desires.

For once—sometimes for the very first time in their lives—these kids get to be in control.

If the wish is farther away, another chapter may meet the family and escort them on their wish, whether it's shopping, celebrity meet-and-greets, or other adventures.

When wish kids come to our area, we're sometimes asked to help on last-minute events, like celebrity greetings. I've been lucky to escort families to concerts, dinners, and backstage meetups, gaining immense respect for the stars who treat wish families with such kindness.

I jump on meet-and-greet opportunities for many reasons, but mostly because I connect deeply with kids who want to meet their favorite celebrity. It doesn't matter who the celebrity is. Honestly, I'd travel anywhere to help grant a wish to meet Johnny Depp (or Lana Parrilla). I'd spoil that child with films and merchandise they never knew they needed. *Sigh. Anyway ...*

What fascinates me is the story behind why that child chose that particular celebrity. It's never just a whim. These celebrities often hold a special place in the child's heart—they helped them get through treatment or their illness. Maybe listening to an artist's music helped during radiation. Maybe watching a sports team's games was how they passed infusion hours. Maybe a TV show allowed them to experience nature or joy when they couldn't go outside to play. Or maybe an actor's work was the only thing that helped them forget the pain for a little while or heal emotionally.

Celebrities, without even realizing it, change lives worldwide by bringing joy and comfort across language and cultural barriers. It takes a special kind of person to step beyond that and actively grant a child's wish. I have endless respect for those who go out of their way for wish kids.

When it comes to Disney World wishes, the magic continues well beyond the wish itself. Families stay at an incredible resort designed just for them—Give Kids the World Village. Only families with children facing critical illnesses on a Make-A-Wish or through a similar organization stay there.

The suites are designed for comfort, and every aspect of the resort caters to the kids. There's ice cream pretty much all day long, an accessible carousel, a giant Candy Land playground, pools and water play areas, and much more. It's fully handicap accessible and offers special events every day—parties, holiday celebrations, character meet-and-greets …

Most of the day-to-day work is done by volunteers—some regulars, some one-time helpers.

When my family went to Disney one year—something we saved for and tried to do every few years—I carved out time to volunteer at Give Kids the World. I wanted to see it for myself, to speak from firsthand experience about how magnificent it is, and because I wanted to give back to this important part of the wish process.

Some kids have told me they don't even want to leave the resort because it feels just as magical—sometimes even better—than the parks themselves. The hardest part is getting there, because it's far enough away that you can't use the regular Disney transportation, so you need to arrange alternate travel.

Luckily, one of the wish families I'd helped with their Disney wish the previous year was going back at the same time and also wanted to volunteer. We arranged to work the same shift, and they gave me a ride. That full-circle moment, volunteering alongside those strong, inspiring people, was a highlight of my trip.

Even cooler was bumping into a current wish family at Give Kids the World while volunteering. I connected with them in the dining hall—my first time meeting a family during their wish trip. It was incredibly special.

Long before I volunteered with Make-A-Wish—before I even imagined helping grant wishes—I was deep in treatment, processing everything my own way. During one of those long hospital stays, I began writing what would become my first children's book: *Thumper's Hospital Adventure*.

It started as simple drawings—which I'm terrible at— and daydreams about what Thumper would do in the middle of the night while I was asleep. It was a fun, personal project, but I had bigger plans.

I kept seeing cancer represented in books and movies in such unrealistic, sensationalized ways. The cancer patient was often fragile and usually died. There were few stories that inspired me as a patient, and no "normal" children's books that accurately portrayed the disease. So, I decided Thumper would be the character to give me the book I wished I had. If the story I needed wasn't out there, I figured it was a sign to create it myself.

Thumper's Hospital Adventure went through a few versions before I realized it was a picture book and I needed an illustrator (because, *seriously*, I cannot draw). The story is told from Thumper's perspective—a toy bunny separated from his best friend Katie (named after me, thanks to my publisher's suggestion) when she is diagnosed with leukemia and admitted to a children's hospital.

Thumper stops at nothing to be by her side again. Along the way, readers learn a little about leukemia and hospitals. The story has a happy ending (spoiler alert), but it also gently acknowledges that not all endings are happy. The comfort comes through the toy bunny's eyes, which makes it relatable because most kids have a favorite plushie in the hospital.

This is a "normal" children's book that any child can enjoy, whether or not they've been affected by cancer or hospitals.

Bringing Thumper's story to life was a meaningful challenge—one that grew far beyond my own journey and became a way to give back. This book is bigger than me (though technically smaller—8.5 by 11 inches—but metaphorically so much larger). I wanted other kids to see themselves accurately represented in an everyday children's book. Every penny from the book's proceeds goes to Make-A-Wish to help children around the world get their wish.

I can never repay Make-A-Wish for changing my life, but this is my way to say thank you.

The book is dedicated to Thumper and Johnny Depp, because both helped me through treatment. Johnny somehow found the book and sent me the most precious note, telling me how touched he was. I may have cried … a lot.

Encouraged by the success of the first book, I felt motivated to continue Thumper's story with a new adventure inspired by my Make-A-Wish experience. I like the idea of teaching readers something quietly—this book teaches Roman numerals, reading analog clocks, and London landmarks.

The second book is *Thumper's London Adventure*. I was lucky to have my illustrator and friend help publish it within four years of the first—a quick turnaround, especially considering we both had full-time jobs and COVID happened in the middle.

I had the crazy idea to ask Johnny Depp to write a foreword. Proceeds would go to Make-A-Wish again, and I wanted some other perspective on why the organization matters. I can say all I want, but who am I to explain it fully?

Asking Johnny felt like a long shot (I even talked myself out of it before sending the request), but he's an unbelievable person and said yes.

So *Thumper's London Adventure* features a heartfelt foreword by my hero, Johnny Depp. When the book was published, it renewed interest in the first one, and Make-A-Wish had an outstanding year. I hope to keep that going for years to come.

I have a crazy dream (I have many) of someday helping donate a million dollars to Make-A-Wish—maybe after a few more books or when *Thumper* becomes a movie. ;)

Despite all the hardships, I've learned to find silver linings and unexpected strength. No one wants to hear they have cancer, and I hope for a day when it's eradicated and no one fears those words again. Until then, I find comfort knowing that even the darkest clouds have silver linings, and good things can come out of terrible events.

You won't be the same after a diagnosis. You must find a new normal. The process can be messy and tumultuous, but the result can surpass your expectations. I have several lumps to prove what I've been through, but overall, I'm a better, stronger person.

Cancer changed my life—but I get to decide what I do with that change. And I choose to make it matter.

Chapter 10
Conclusion & Last Thoughts

Congratulations! You've made it to the final chapter of this book. Unless, of course, you skipped ahead—then congrats on finding the end.

While memory and cognitive struggles were constant hurdles throughout my journey, they weren't the only ones. When treatment ended, new challenges emerged—like navigating relationships and deciding how much of my story to share. Do I tell someone I'm a survivor right away? Does this history make me somehow damaged or broken? Should I seek a partner who's also a survivor?

I chose to be upfront. Any potential partner would know from the beginning. If they couldn't handle it, they weren't worth my time. Having had cancer isn't something I could change about myself, so why pretend it didn't happen?

I'll never forget mentioning it to my now-husband on our first date. He didn't flinch. Now, did he know what kind of baggage I came with? Probably not. But who really knows everything about someone after a first date, anyway? I'm not even sure if I knew his last name …

For many, hearing someone is a cancer survivor can feel intimidating—or even be a deal breaker. Even when it's in your past, it becomes part of the foundation your future is built on. You can't erase that reality. And while no one can guarantee they'll never face cancer, knowing it's already in the picture is a different kind of choice.

Because cancer doesn't happen in isolation. One person may carry the diagnosis, but it affects their entire circle— their family, their friends, their caregivers. It's a shared burden, even if the physical weight rests on just one set of shoulders.

It's hard having cancer. You watch your friends live normal lives while your future hangs in the balance. Your family tries to carry on, pretending their world isn't falling apart. You see fellow patients you've grown to love lose their battles, and you keep going, all the while fearing you might leave your own family grieving. Parents without a child. A brother without his sister.

I had cancer—and I was living it every day—but sometimes I forgot that my family was living it, too.

Cancer touches more than just the patient. It quietly reshapes the lives of everyone who loves them. I can only imagine how powerless my family must have felt. I always knew how I was feeling (well, more or less). I had some control over how I responded emotionally. But they? They had to watch. They had little say in the outcome. Looking back, if given the choice between being sick or being in their position—I think I'd choose to be the patient every time. I'd never want to put them through what I went through physically … and I certainly wouldn't want to endure the helplessness they must have felt.

In hindsight, I wish I'd gone to therapy during treatment. (I may have mentioned that once or ten times.) At the time, I thought, "What could a stranger possibly say that would help?" I didn't believe anyone could truly understand what I was facing. But talking might have helped. Instead, I vented to the people closest to me—probably more than they could handle at times. I'll always be grateful to the friends, family, and teachers who listened, who showed up, and who carried what they could of my pain.

Humor was my armor. My coping mechanism of choice. Even when it wasn't appropriate (especially then). I remember a teacher once warned us about something being dangerous, and my knee-jerk response, full of sass, was: "What'll it do—give me cancer?" Without skipping a beat, the teacher reminded me that I could still develop *other* cancers. (A fun little fact I get to live with: the possibility of secondary cancers thanks to treatment. And I might not be so lucky next time.)

I needed that teacher. I needed people who could lovingly call me out, help keep me grounded, and stop me from spiraling into dark places. People who could hold space for the heavy while reminding me that my life wasn't over.

Because facing cancer meant facing mortality head-on—something most people avoid until absolutely necessary.

Coming to terms with your own mortality might be one of life's most challenging mental and emotional tasks. When you're told you might die sooner than expected, it's like being enrolled in an intensive course on human fragility. And even those who are "terminal" might still struggle to believe it. It's a heavy weight to carry at any age—but especially when you're young. No child—or their family—should have to deal with that kind of reality.

I won't pretend I'm ready to die. But cancer forced me to accept that I won't live forever, and that awareness has pushed me to live more intentionally.

It wasn't a straight line to acceptance. In the beginning, my diagnosis felt like a curse—a single event that shattered everything. I hated the day it happened. I blamed it for ruining my life. (Let's be honest: who *hasn't* been dramatically bitter at some point?) But after a lot of healing, soul-searching, and growth, I started to see the unexpected blessings that followed.

Now, every year on my "cancerversary," my family celebrates. Not because we're happy I had cancer, but because we recognize what that day has brought us: perspective, appreciation, and another year together—something no one is guaranteed.

Sometimes I wonder: if I could go back and erase November 14, 2007—the day I was diagnosed—would I do it? If I could have remained a healthy teenager, would I?

It's a strange thought experiment. Would I trade everything I've experienced just to avoid the pain?

I don't have a clear answer. And maybe that's okay.

Sure, on the surface, it sounds like an obvious "yes." Who wouldn't want to skip the trauma of cancer? But then

… cancer shaped me. It changed the trajectory of my life. It introduced me to people, places, and parts of myself I might never have known otherwise. I like the woman I am today. I'm not sure I would have liked the version of me that would have grown up untouched by this path.

Yes, I'll always live with the risks—late effects, potential infertility, the looming chance of recurrence or secondary cancers. I may not live as long as others. But I'm here now. And I've learned not to waste too much time on "what ifs."

Living with uncertainty is just part of the deal now. But honestly, can any of us fully untangle the impact of one life event from all the rest? Who's to say which parts of my life came from cancer and which would have happened anyway?

Would I have gotten involved with Make-A-Wish if I'd always been healthy? Would I have fallen in love with London otherwise? Would I have met my husband—someone I first connected with over our mutual love of London (and Disney)? Would I have published *Thumper's Adventures*? Or written this memoir? Would I ever have met Johnny Depp?

Probably not.

And without those pieces … who would I even be? I'll never know—and honestly, I'm grateful for that.

So, did I avoid answering the question I asked myself? Maybe. But if I had to choose … I probably wouldn't change anything.

Whatever trials you've faced—or are facing—I hope you grow from them.

I hope you spend time with those you love.

And I hope you find every silver lining, even if it takes time and a little squinting to see it.

Acknowledgments

First and foremost, to my parents and my brother, D.J.— thank you for being my constants through the chaos. Your love, strength, and food runs did not go unnoticed.

To Jay—thank you for turning my stories (and this cover) into art, and for making illustrations of Thumper look cuter than I ever could've imagined. Speaking of: Thumper, my forever sidekick—you've been with me through it all, with your stylish sweaters and unwavering support.

To the amazing teachers who didn't just teach, but truly *showed up*—especially my Chemistry teacher, who made science lessons and chemo compatible. You fueled the spark that led me to the classroom.

To Lisa Lee, my editor, for your thoughtful suggestions to help me polish my thoughts.

To the brilliant doctors, nurses, and all my extended family at CCMC—you made a terrifying time survivable, even laughable at times. To my teen group and all who cancer brought into my life—thank you for the friendships, the resilience, and the perspective.

To Cory, for motivating me to write this (and not allowing me to give up when I wanted to). I hope more people in similar situations tell their stories and that others can benefit from and be inspired by them.

To those this disease took—especially the ones mentioned in this memoir—you are deeply missed and forever an integral part of my journey.

To everyone who supported my family through this journey, in big ways and small—even if we didn't take you up on the offer, your kindness was seen and felt.

To everyone at Make-A-Wish, and to those who played a part in granting my wish—thank you for reminding me that magic still exists.

To Johnny Depp—your talent and kindness not only helped me through treatment but inspired me to give back and grow in ways I never imagined.

To Lana Parrilla—though you came into my life after treatment, your work helped me face and heal wounds I didn't fully realize I was still carrying.

To my husband, Jake—thank you for walking into this story long after treatment ended, but still choosing to love me every day and help shoulder the aftermath with me. That means everything.

To everyone facing this disease in any capacity or fighting their own battles. You are seen. You are stronger than you can even imagine. Keep going.

And to everyone mentioned or alluded to in this book— thank you for being a part of my story.

With love,

Katie

Now What?

If you're reading this, there's a good chance cancer has already touched your life in a very real way. Maybe you're in the middle of it. Maybe you're on the other side, still figuring out what "after" looks like. Maybe you care about someone who's fighting—or who fought—and you may be wondering: *What can I do?* Whatever brought you here, you're not alone.

This book is my story of growing up with cancer. I survived, and today I am okay (*knock on wood*). Some moments in these pages may seem small or trivial on the surface, but they mattered deeply at the time. I share them for teens, young adults, and caregivers walking—or still carrying—a similar journey, in the hope that they feel seen and less alone.

A portion of the proceeds from this book is donated to support childhood cancer research. But money is only one way forward—and for many families walking this road, it may not be the right way at the moment.

Progress in childhood cancer treatment didn't happen by accident. It happened because patients, families, researchers, and advocates refused to stay silent—because people shared their stories, pushed for better options, and believed survival could look different than it did before.

That work isn't finished.

Thinking beyond ourselves doesn't always mean giving more. Sometimes it means speaking up. Sometimes it means telling our truth. Sometimes it simply means reminding the next family or cancer patient that they're not facing this alone.

If and when you're able, you may wish to learn more about organizations supporting childhood cancer research and advocacy. The following is a non-exhaustive list—just places to begin your own search:

- St. Jude Children's Research Hospital
- National Pediatric Cancer Foundation (NPCF)
- Alex's Lemonade Stand Foundation (ALSF)
- Pediatric Cancer Research Foundation (PCRF)
- Rally Foundation for Childhood Cancer Research
- CureSearch for Children's Cancer
- Children's Cancer Research Fund (CCRF)

Each supports childhood cancer research in different ways, from funding science to amplifying patient voices. Even small contributions—of money, time, or attention—matter.

If this book gave you language for something you've lived through, consider sharing your story when you're ready. If it reminded you of how far we've come, consider advocating for how much further we still need to go. If it simply made you feel a little less alone, that matters too.

Survival is not the end of the story; it's the beginning. And the story gets better when more of us are willing to tell it.

Thank you for reading. And thank you for caring enough to take the next step.

www.ingramcontent.com/pod-product-compliance
Lightning Source LLC
Chambersburg PA
CBHW072046150726

47996CB00015B/1687